CORRECTING THE VITAMIN D DEFICIENCY EPIDEMIC

Strategies to Fight Diseases and Prolong Life for Black People

Emily Allison-Francis, M.S., M.L.S.,
Post Grad. Dip. Ed.

5/31/12
Bro Austin Truth
Peace & Love

DARE BOOKS
Orlando, FL

Francis

Author's Note

This book is in essence a compilation of the author's opinions, beliefs and ideas, based on her educational background and her analysis of relevant resources relating to the subject matter covered within its pages. It is the author's intent to provide you, the reader, with fresh and nuanced perspectives and analyses that will expand your knowledge base, enrich your understanding and peak your interest to learn more. In doing so, however, the author wants to make it abundantly clear to the reader that because the information covered in this book is seminal in many respects, and is based on the author's opinions and independent analysis and interpretation of the resource materials available to her at the time of publication, it should be relied upon solely as a supplemental information resource and should not, under any circumstance be considered to be, or used in lieu of, professional medical advice. The author is not, and does not profess to be, a medical doctor and this book is being made available to you with the understanding that neither the author nor the publisher is engaging in rendering professional medical, health, or other personal professional services via this book. Furthermore, because this book is to be used solely for supplemental informational purposes and should not be construed as medical advice, your reading this book does not in any way replace the need for obtaining the advice of, or seeking a medical evaluation from, a physician. An in-person consultation with a competent medical professional who has the opportunity to assess your individual health history and situation is invaluable, and should not be discounted or taken for granted. You are strongly encouraged to check with your doctor before following any recommendations, adopting any of the suggestions or drawing inferences from any information contained in this book and definitely before self-treating any condition that may require medical diagnosis or attention. The author and publisher of this book specifically disclaim any responsibility to you, or any other person or persons directly or indirectly affected by your reliance on information contained in this book.

Library of Congress Cataloging-in-Publication Data

Allison-Francis, Emily.
    Correcting the vitamin D deficiency epidemic: strategies to fight diseases and prolong life for black people / Emily Allison-Francis.
        p. cm.
    Includes bibliographical references and index
    ISBN 978-0-912444-49-9 (alk. paper)
1. Vitamin D in human nutrition—Popular works. 2. Vitamin D deficiency—Popular works.
3. African Americans—Health and hygiene—Popular works. I. Title.
    QP772.V53A45 2011
    612.3'99—dc23
                            2011030004
            Index by Clive Pyne Indexing Services
            Printed in Canada

To
my parents Nerissa and Aquilla Allison whose guiding spirit serves as my inspiration for persevering. Their memory sparked my motivation and energized me during the years that I spent writing this book

and
my many friends and relatives who died from chronic vitamin D related illnesses before they could benefit from the groundbreaking research on vitamin D.

Contents

Acknowledgments

I am grateful to the students of Medgar Evers College of the City University of New York for the opportunity to receive their research queries and to direct their database searches. Many of these searches often led to eye-opening discoveries, showing the disproportionate disease and mortality rates among dark-skinned people. These issues served as a springboard for the writing of this book.

Thanks to Professor Vanrea Thomas, my mentor and chief librarian at Medgar Evers College of the City University of New York. My research skills were sharpened by the many information literacy and research training sessions that Professor Thomas held with the library staff.

This book would not be possible without the groundbreaking research of Vitamin D scientists in the United States of America and other parts of the world. I have tremendous appreciation for their work which has helped to make a difference in so many people's lives. I owe a wealth of gratitude to Dr. William Grant and other members of the *Vitamin D Council* for their pioneering work in establishing the critical importance of vitamin D to good health. I also thank Dr. Grant for his thoughtful and constructive comments about this book.

I thank Dr. Gerald Deas, Associate Professor of Medicine, State University of New York, for being a pioneer in the field of preventive medicine for many years and for his valuable suggestions and recommendations.

Dr. Mitzi Reid has been our family physician for more than 20 years. I am grateful to her for writing the foreword for this book.

Heartfelt thanks go to my brother McNal, my nephew Shawn, and my colleagues Sebert Harper and Cristelin Henry for their steadfast encouragement and kind assistance.

My deepest appreciation goes to my husband Orville, and my children, Tricia, Tamara, and Paul, for their unwavering love and support. I am also extremely thankful for the excellent insights they offered and the invaluable editorial assistance they provided throughout the writing of this book. Thank you all for taking this journey with me.

Foreword

Dr. Mitzi A. Reid

Correcting the Vitamin D Deficiency Epidemic: Strategies to Fight Diseases and Prolong Life for Black People is a timely book that addresses the unique vitamin D needs of dark-skinned people. Health statistics show that blacks suffer disproportionately from major chronic diseases such as high blood pressure, heart disease, diabetes and cancer, which are associated with vitamin D deficiency. Many blacks are simply not aware of their unique vitamin D needs and that many of the chronic diseases from which they suffer can be greatly reduced if their vitamin D levels are normalized. In this book Emily Francis explains the health enhancing and, in many instances, life-saving qualities of vitamin D, especially for dark-skinned people.

Conventional medicine has not done a very good job of emphasizing the critically important role that vitamin D plays in establishing and maintaining good health. Perhaps more importantly, dark-skinned people are simply not being told by their doctors that they have unique vitamin D needs because high melanin concentrations in their skin inhibit vitamin D production from the sun. Consequently, dark-skinned people need to spend far more time in the sun than whites if they want to make sufficient amounts of vitamin D. Supplementation with vitamin D is quite often necessary for dark-skinned people because they simply cannot make enough vitamin D if they are not getting adequate sun exposure.

I applaud the author for emphasizing the importance of adequate vitamin D levels in pregnant black women and young children. Pregnant black women, who are usually critically deficient in vitamin D, often pass on their vitamin D deficiency status to their children. Many diseases that are diagnosed later in life such as cancer, diabetes, and auto-immune diseases, are often associated with early childhood vitamin D deficiency.

As a practicing primary care physician, I have seen marked improvement in my patients' health when their vitamin D levels are normalized. The author also highlights the importance of eating nutrient-rich foods and regular, effective exercise for creating and maintaining good health. The recommendations in this book can improve the health and well-being of many people and save many lives as well. It should be required reading for all health care practitioners and certainly for all blacks.

Introduction

Black people[1] in the United States of America are sicker and are dying from major chronic diseases at a much higher rate than their white counterparts. Not only do blacks suffer from more major illnesses but they also have lower survival rates and die at a younger age than whites.[2] Cultural habits and economic conditions are often blamed for the higher disease and mortality rates among blacks. However, this reasoning does not pass the scrutiny test when viewed in light of groundbreaking research on the correlation between vitamin D deficiency and chronic diseases and the high rate of vitamin D deficiency in blacks relative to whites.

A review of relevant literature on vitamin D shows dire health consequences from vitamin D deficiency. Some studies have noted that dark-skinned people are more susceptible to being deficient in vitamin D. However, to date, no major study has established a comprehensive link between the critically low vitamin D status of most blacks and the alarmingly high rates of chronic disease and mortality in the black population. This book fills a crucial void in the scientific literature on the role of vitamin D in disease control and prevention by establishing a connection between the critical vitamin D deficiency status of most blacks and the skyrocketing rates of disease and mortality among blacks.

Skyrocketing Rates of Illness Among Blacks

Statistics have shown that blacks are disproportionately affected by cancer and other chronic diseases. Inflammatory

---

[1] The terms "black" and "blacks" are used throughout this book as phenotypic descriptors for dark pigmented persons of all ancestries.

[2] The terms "white" and "whites" are used throughout this book as phenotypic descriptors for light pigmented persons of all ancestries.

1

diseases seem to be reducing the quality and life expectancy of blacks. The HIV/AIDS crisis is a prime example. According to the United States Centers for Disease Control and Prevention (CDC), more than half a million blacks have been diagnosed with AIDS since the outset of the AIDS epidemic in the United States. In the United States, although they account for 12 percent of the United States population, blacks make up almost fifty percent of new AIDS cases. Black women account for two thirds of these cases. This is about sixteen times the rate of infection in white women. HIV kills blacks in disproportionate numbers and affects young black females at an alarming rate.

Misguided Assumptions about Blacks

It is a commonly held belief that lifestyle practices and socioeconomic conditions make blacks unhealthy. African Americans have been found to have lower life expectancy than white Americans and statistics show that blacks are about three times more likely to die from the ten leading causes of death. Many have attributed these findings to low income levels, inadequate access to health care, and limited access to fresh fruits and vegetables in poor, predominantly black communities. However, despite having better access to healthcare than poor blacks, middle class black professionals also suffer higher rates of chronic diseases than whites.

While poor education and lack of healthy food choices contribute greatly to ill-health, and even death, I submit that the disproportionate rate of disease and mortality among blacks has more to do with the fact that dark-skinned people are especially prone to being chronically deficient in vitamin D, a vital health enhancing nutrient. This book will hopefully help to dispel the widely held belief that socioeconomic and cultural factors are the main reasons for higher disease and mortality rates among blacks and show that the disproportionately high rates of disease and mortality among blacks are due in large part to serious deficiency in the critical nutrient, vitamin D.

Dispelling the Myth – The Melanin Factor

A study done on a New York City community provides health data that help dispel the myth that socio-cultural practices are the major contributing factor to the high rates of chronic illness among blacks. This New York City community has a population of 316,000 with approximately 80 percent blacks. This community has more college educated residents and high school graduates, higher average income, and more green grocery stores than the neighboring communities that are predominantly white. Nonetheless, black residents in this community suffer more from major chronic diseases than the neighboring white communities. How do we explain this? I suggest that critically high rates of vitamin D deficiency among dark-skinned people is largely responsible for the high rates of chronic disease in this New York City community. This dire situation affects darkly pigmented people worldwide.

Dark skin pigmentation preserves folate stores for successful reproduction, protects from early aging of the skin, and helps prevent skin cancer caused from over exposure to the ultraviolet rays of the sun, but it also hinders sunlight from entering the skin. This inhibits production of vitamin D, the nutrient that helps prevent dozens of diseases. Dark skin pigmentation in blacks predisposes them to chronic vitamin D deficiency and results in significantly higher rates of disease and mortality in the black population. However, with adequate supplementation dark-skinned people can correct their vitamin D deficiency and help prevent major chronic diseases.

You will find the information in this book useful for helping you and your family maintain optimum health and prevent diseases. Reading this book will hopefully help you to become more aware of the unique vitamin D needs of dark-skinned people and the importance of vitamin D and wholesome foods in maintaining good health. The book is divided into two sections. The first part discusses vitamin D deficiency and some of the diseases associated with that deficiency which disproportionately afflict dark-pigmented people. The second part discusses some of the many benefits of eating nutrient-rich, whole foods, resources for finding chemical-free foods, and recipes that will help you prevent and reverse many disease conditions.

PART ONE

The Wonder-Working Functions of Vitamin D

Chapter 1

Rays of Life

The sun contains more than 99 percent of the mass of the planetary system and sustains life on earth. The sun is a star and it stands fixed in the center of eight heavenly bodies known as planets. The planets rotate on their axes as they revolve around the sun. The earth's rotation on its axis gives us day and night, and its movement around the sun gives the seasons of the year with varied intensity of sunlight, different degrees of ultraviolet radiation (UVR), and various life-enhancing photoproducts. Our primary source of heat on earth comes from radiation from the sun and without this radiation life would not exist on earth. Sunlight emerges as a wonder among the majestic forces of creation.

Mother nature ensures that when you expose your body to the sun, you get vitamin D and as many as ten other biological photoproducts. There is nothing like the real thing. It is difficult to overdose on vitamin D from supplements, but if you take extremely high doses for an extended period of time you could develop toxicity. It is not like this with sun exposure. You will not overdose on vitamin D from sun exposure. Your body has a built-in regulator that controls vitamin D production from the sun. Vitamin D made in the skin by the sun lasts about twice as long as vitamin D that you ingest from food or supplements. Nonetheless, sunlight may not always be available or you may not be able to spend enough time in the sun. In these cases, you need to take vitamin D supplements, especially if your skin pigmentation is dark.

Various human activities are directly affected by the sun's rays. Seasonal planting of crops and harvesting are only a few of these activities. Epidemics, patterns of conception and birth, birth weight and acute attacks from diseases such as asthma and heart attacks, depression and seasonal affective disorder (SAD) are all influenced by the sun and seasons of the year. Vitamin D production from the sun plays an indispensable role in preserving life and health.

Sunlight and the Grand Design of Life

The benefits of sunlight are as myriad as they are indispensable. Sunlight is an essential part of the processes that produce oxygen and food in the earth's ecosystems. Sunlight disinfects water for consumption, cures skin diseases, builds sturdy stems in plants, and reduces germination of spores that cause allergies from which so many people suffer. Both plants and animals have biological organs that help them to make use of sunlight in their respective environments. Diseases are more prevalent when the sun's ultraviolet B (UVB) rays are limited and vitamin D production from the sun is low.

Our very existence depends on the sun because sunlight is an integral part of the processes that sustain life on our planet. The sun's rays stream continuously and provide substances that cover the earth and invigorate life. Plants and animals need solar energy, but animals, including humans, use this energy after it is captured and transformed by green plants. Rays of the sun get onto the leaves of green plants and plants capture this solar energy through a process called photosynthesis. Green plants carry out photosynthesis and this process produces the fruits and vegetables we eat and oxygen in the air that we breathe. Plants are producers because they harvest sunlight and use it to produce food, making possible the various food chains and food webs that sustain life on land and in oceans, seas, and rivers. The production of the wonder hormone, vitamin D, bears striking similarity to the production of food and oxygen - the products of photosynthesis.

Sunlight and Your Sleep/Wake Pattern

Sunlight affects the daily ebb and flow of hormones in your body, and your hormones affect your sleep pattern, appetite, energy levels, mood, and your ability to think and act. When night falls, the hypothalamus, a gland that is deeply buried in your brain, sends a signal to the pineal gland in your brain. The pineal gland got its name from its resemblance to a tiny pine cone but this gland has immense effect on your emotional and physical wellbeing. The pineal gland releases a substance called melatonin. Melatonin makes your system wind down so that you are prepared to sleep at nights, a function that is essential for your health.

When day breaks, the photoreceptors in the retina of your eye receive light signals and send these signals along the optic nerve at the back of your eye to the hypothalamus of your brain. The hypothalamus gland, buried deeply in your brain, integrates a huge mass of data and sends a different set of information to the pineal gland. This time, information from the hypothalamus stimulates the pineal gland to shut down the production of melatonin, the sleep hormone, and increase production of serotonin, the "feel good" hormone which makes you alert. If there is a malfunction in your melatonin/serotonin production mechanism, you may wake feeling groggy and depressed.

Your sleep/wake pattern is healthy when you wake up feeling alert and in good spirits. Scientists continue to discover how sunlight affects your body clock and how food nutrients and your sleep environment can help you to get more restful sleep at nights. There are many health factors that may affect your ability to get a good night's sleep. However, when you spend more time in the sun and have adequate amounts of vitamin D, calcium and magnesium in your body, your biological sleep clock functions even better.

Some Sunglasses Can Cause Depression

Some sunglasses can raise your blood melatonin level during the day and cause you to be depressed. Blue tinted sunglasses prevent blue light from entering your eyes. Blue light from the sun enters the retina of your eye and travels via the optic nerve in the back of your eye to your brain. Under normal conditions, this light stimulates your hypothalamus and pineal glands to reduce the production of melatonin and increase production of serotonin. When you wear sunglasses that block the rays of the sun, the glands in your brain produce more melatonin, the sleep hormone, and less serotonin, the awake or feel-good hormone. Keep the blue tinted sunglasses off and experience the mood-boosting effect of sunlight that is absorbed through your eye.

Sunlight Reduces Germination of Spores That Cause Allergies

Environmental allergens have the potential to affect every-one but sunlight reduces the ability of spores to germinate. If you have an allergy that bothers you constantly, especially when seasons change, you may be allergic to spores that are dispersed in the air by molds or other fungi. Molds and mildew are fungi that often grow in dark damp places such as basements, bath-rooms, and kitchens. However, molds live everywhere and they disperse their spores in the air. Wind spreads spores of molds in indoor as well as outdoor air, and inhaling the spores can cause allergic reactions.

Mold spores are very resilient but sunlight can be used to reduce their germination. One study reported on in a 2003 issue of *Granna*, notes that sunlight decreased spore germination of *Alternaria alternata,* a mold associated with irritation of the upper respiratory tract and gut, from 85 percent to 5 percent. Exposure to this mold increases one's chances of attacks from asthma. The study also found that metabolic activities of the spores declined by 34 percent in the presence of sunlight. This mold is often found indoors on carpets, textiles, window frames, and damp dark places. Now we have good reason for letting the sunshine in and occasionally sunning our rugs and carpets. Getting adequate sunlight exposure might also deactivate some of the harmful spores that we carry around on our bodies.

Sunlight Destroys Harmful Bacteria in Water

Contaminated water is an important health issue because pathogens in water are associated with infection of the gastrointestinal tract, respiratory tract, urinary tract, joints, bone and skin. Disease causing pathogens such as bacteria are often found in water used for drinking and household purposes, but sunlight can be used to kill these pathogens. This natural way of disinfecting water is cost effective and environmentally friendly. While killing waterborne bacteria, sunlight can also break apart dangerous chemicals in water. A study published in a 2010 issue of *Photochemistry and Photobiology* reports that sunlight can be used to damage the outer membrane of bacteria leading to death of the bacteria.

The antibacterial property of sunlight holds much significance for public health in developing countries as well as in more industrialized countries. A large percentage of illnesses in children and adults in developing countries is caused from waterborne viruses, bacteria and protozoa. Very young children, sick, and elderly people are especially susceptible to waterborne pathogens. Water that contains dangerous micro-organisms can lead to diseases such as tuberculosis, hepatitis B, meningitis, typhoid fever, cholera, poliomyelitis, and other diseases. We sometimes hear about outbreaks of these diseases in developing countries but water sources in more industrialized countries such as the U.S. are also susceptible to these outbreaks. For example, E. coli bacteria (bacteria in human feces) sometimes get channeled into drinking water, and foods sold in the U.S. are sometimes infected with E. coli bacteria.

When found in water, the E. coli species can be easily inactivated by ultraviolet light rays that are found in the natural spectrum of the sun. In one method of purifying water, an ultraviolet lamp is used to capture ultraviolet radiation passing the rays on to water in a flow chamber. The water absorbs the rays from the lamp and ultraviolet energy gets transmitted into the structures of the viruses, and cells of bacteria in the water.

This process destroys the pathogens and removes the risk of getting disease from the water.

Municipalities often treat water with chemical additives in order to render it safe for drinking. However, solar radiation may be an easier and safer way to purify water. Scientists say that when adequately clean water in a sealed, transparent container is placed in the sun for 6 or more hours, UV radiation kills pathogens so that the water becomes potable. There are additional benefits to using sunlight to disinfect water. This method of disinfecting water does not remove beneficial minerals. Neither does it affect the taste and odor of water. Additionally, the cost effectiveness and environmentally friendly nature of sunlight purification gives this method an important place in the current green revolution. Sunlight purification of water may prove an invaluable method for people who obtain their drinking water from untreated sources. Solar radiation of water will therefore be beneficial to impoverished communities because the materials used for it are usually readily available in these communities at minimal or no cost. As you can imagine, you need to start the UV purification process using minimally safe water, with no dangerous chemicals or macroscopic matter floating in it.

Increased Sun Exposure Helps Skin Problems

Sunlight helps the body to destroy internal disease agents as well as pathogens that anchor themselves on the surface of the skin. The skin is often colonized by parasites and people of all ages may suffer from skin infection. However, young children and the elderly tend to have sensitive skin types and are therefore more vulnerable to getting bacterial and fungal infections of the skin.

Adequate sun exposure has been found to have a positive effect on some skin disorders such as atopic eczema. One study published in a 2006 publication of the journal *Allergy,* notes that Norwegian children suffering from atopic eczema saw significant reductions in their condition when they were taken to the Canary Islands, a sunlight rich region, off the northern coast of Africa.

Sunlight Regulates Plant Life

Sunlight regulates seed germination, plant growth, flowering, shade avoidance response mechanisms in plants and the length of plant life. A seed contains enough food to support the emergence of the young plant from the seed, but after emerging the new plant needs sunlight to grow. From this stage until the end of its life cycle, a plant uses sunlight to carry out various physiological activities.

The seedling uses sunlight to carry out photosynthesis and this process provides food that the seedling needs to grow. UVB radiation from the sun can alter the timing of flowering and the number of flowers in many plant species. This also affects production of fruits. Agricultural scientists and farmers plant crops according to sunlight hours and seasons of the year because they know that sunlight has a powerful effect on crop production. Sunlight also helps to build sturdy stems in plants and sturdy stems facilitate better transport of plant food from roots to the leaves of plants. Plants demonstrate a principle of the great design of nature when they grow towards sunlight.

Sunlight-Rich Regions

You may completely take for granted the health sustaining benefits of the sun despite living in a sunlight rich region. You may also be suffering from inadequate sunlight exposure in the midst of abundant sunshine. If you work indoors you need to find some time to expose your skin to the abundant sunshine in your environment. Doctors in sunny California have expressed surprise about the low levels of vitamin D in many of their patients who live there.

Whether you live in sun-drenched or sun-deprived areas, it is crucially important that you get the amount of sunshine your body needs. The only way to do this is to get in the sun and be sure to spend approximately three hours each day if you are dark-skinned. If sunshine is unavailable, you should substitute by taking vitamin D supplements. This will provide you with some of the sun's health enhancing nutrients. Sunshine saves hundreds of thousands of lives each year. A light-skinned person needs about twenty minutes of sun exposure per day to manufacture enough vitamin D, while a dark-skinned person needs to be in the sun for approximately three hours daily to produce a similar amount of vitamin D. This is approximately 3,000 IU of vitamin D. Vitamin D scientists believe that a healthy adult should take about 5,000 IU of vitamin D each day, but dark-skinned people may need to take more in order to optimize their vitamin D levels.

Latitude and Vitamin D Production

The earth is a sphere that has measurements called lines of latitude. These imaginary lines are drawn on world maps and they encircle the earth and run parallel to the equator, north and south of the equator. Lines of latitude running north of the equator denote the northern hemisphere and those running south of the equator identify the southern hemisphere. North latitude lines measure the distance, in degrees, north of the equator while south latitude lines measure distance, also in degrees, south of the equator. For ease of reference, positions of places are stated in degrees of latitude. For example, Chicago is located at 41 degrees north latitude. The greater the degree of latitude, the lower the intensity of UVB (ultraviolet B) radiation for vitamin D production. If you live in New York City or Newark, New Jersey, at 40 degrees north latitude, you would be in a vitamin D deficiency danger zone.

As you go north of the equator, latitude increases and the rays of the sun pass through more layers of air. This reduces the intensity of ultraviolet light and vitamin D production from the sun. The further from the tropics you go the less direct sunlight you get until the northernmost and southernmost points are reached. At the greatest latitude—the point of the earth furthest away from the equator—the rays of the sun pass through so many layers of air that there is almost no sunshine and living things may not be able to survive. However, large numbers of people, especially blacks, are dying from vitamin D-related diseases in regions with high latitude as well as low latitude. This is because dark-skinned people are not taking time to get their bare skin exposed to two to three hours of sunshine every day, and they are not taking enough vitamin D supplements to compensate for the shortfall in vitamin D when there is little sun exposure.

Health Risks in High Latitude Areas

Studies have shown that northern sunlight does not always contribute to vitamin D production. UVB rays of the sun get through your skin to produce vitamin D, but there is virtually none in winter. This is the case if you live in northern climates such as the United States, Canada, Britain and other European countries. These regions are located above 35 degrees latitude, far away from the equator where the sun shines more directly overhead. In these colder regions, located above 35 degrees latitude, you get about zero vitamin D from the sun between the months of November and March, however long you stay in the sun. In northern cities like New York, Hartford, Boston and Chicago you may have enough vitamin D at the end of summer but by the end of winter your blood vitamin D levels might be depleted. This helps to explain why these regions are said to comprise the cancer belt, multiple sclerosis zone, and asthma epicenters, especially for blacks.

Everyone living in high latitude regions is in danger of being deficient in vitamin D but dark-skinned people are in the greatest danger. A cross-sectional study of 150 persons was done in Minneapolis which has a latitude of 44 degrees. The study participants who lived in the inner city of Minneapolis, had persistent muscle and bone pain and were examined at a primary care health center. All of the African American, East African, Hispanic, and American Indian patients were found to be critically deficient in vitamin D. All of the patients had vitamin D levels that were less than 20ng/ml. Minneapolis is close to the Canadian border, and the reduced sunlight in this area might have caused the dark-skinned patients to be more deficient in vitamin D.

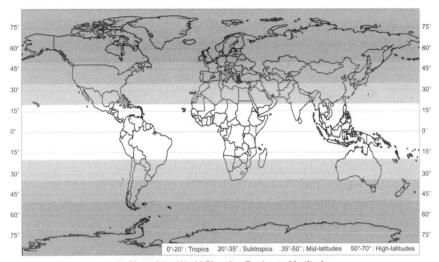

Map of the World Showing Regions of Latitude

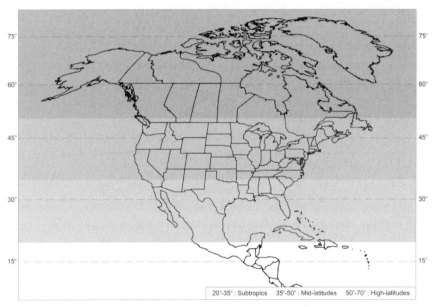

Map of North America Showing Regions of Latitude

High Latitude Cities with Large Black Populations in the United States

City, State	Degrees of Latitude
New York, NJ-NY	41
Chicago, IL	42
Washington, MD-VA	36-39
Nashville, TN	36
Minneapolis-St. Paul, MN	44
Seattle-Tacoma, WA	47
Pittsburgh, PA	40
Philadelphia-Wilmington, PA-DE	39
Detroit, MI	42
Baltimore, MD	39
Memphis, TN	35
San Francisco-Oakland, CA	37
Norfolk, Virginia Beach, VA	36
St. Louis, MO	38
Cleveland, OH	41
Charlotte, NC	35

Raleigh, NC	35
Richmond – Petersburg, VA	37
Boston, MA	42
Hartford, CT	42
New Haven, CT	42
Bridgeport-Stamford, CT	42

Effects of Pollution and Cloud Cover On Vitamin D Production

Atmospheric pollution reduces the intensity of the sun's rays and lowers the production of vitamin D from sunlight. Cloud cover can lower your vitamin D production by half. Urban areas have industrial waste, automobile hydrocarbon and nitric oxide emissions that often cause smog. Smog is toxic to your body and it blocks the rays of the sun. Your vitamin D production from the sun is therefore lower in polluted areas. This has serious implications for blacks. Greater numbers of African Americans live in cities where pollution blocks sunlight and lowers vitamin D. When you live or work in a city or an industrial area, your vitamin D from sunlight is reduced. Dark skin pigmentation further reduces vitamin D production making blacks more vulnerable to diseases.

Cloud cover is formed from droplets of water that are smaller than rain drops. Some regions often carry thick cloud cover and this decreases the intensity of UVB rays, causing vitamin D production from sunlight to be drastically reduced. You can look around you and identify some of the things that inhibit vitamin D production – motor vehicle exhausts, industrial waste from factories, smog, and thick cloud cover.

Your geographic elevation also affects how much UVB you are exposed to. People who live at high elevations have greater access to the rays of the sun that are needed to produce vitamin

D. At lower altitudes or lower elevations, there is less intense ultra-violet radiation from the sun. More rays get absorbed by the atmosphere at higher levels, reducing the quantity of sunlight that is streamed to lower elevations.

Breathing polluted city air may impact your health in negative ways, and if you are dark-skinned the negative effect is greater because you may have less vitamin D to strengthen your immune system. Your vitamin D from the sun's rays might be reduced in intensity because these rays travel through a more polluted atmosphere. However, you may not need to sell your home in the city, give up your apartment or quit your city job to preserve your health. Instead, you can take vitamin D supplements as a necessary health precaution.

Sunlight Cures Anxiety

Sunlight has the power to improve your health in a short period of time. Here is a report from someone who experienced the mood modulating effect of the UVB rays of the sun.

> **Jonathan, a dark-skinned man, living in the Northeastern United States for more than 20 years, explained that he suffered from anxiety. While living in the United States, his doctor prescribed anxiety medication for him but the medication did not alleviate the anxiety symptoms. Jonathan visited the island of Jamaica in the Caribbean, and while there, he assisted with a project that required him to work outdoors for several hours each day. After less than 3 weeks of getting full sun exposure, Jonathan's anxiety symptoms completely disappeared. In Jonathan's words, he was "miraculously healed by the sun." Jonathan experienced the wonder-working power of vitamin D that is produced by the ultraviolet rays of the sun.**

How Much of Your Body Are You Exposing to Sunlight?

It is healthy to sunbathe, so get in your shorts and skinny tops or your bathing suit and allow the rays of the sun to pelt your skin.

When you expose your arms and legs to the sun, 25 percent of your body gets sunlight. Your bare face and the upper region of your chest and back may add another 20 percent of sun exposure. Our clothing prevents different areas of our bodies from getting sun exposure and a great amount of our body is always covered by our clothing. Our bodies are also covered during the long cold seasons in North America. Clothing, along with the melanin in dark skin, blocks sunlight from the body. Many dark-skinned people further endanger their health during summer by applying sunscreen to their bodies.

Sunscreen Lotion Is Bad for Dark-Skinned People

Skin color determines whether you need to use sunscreen lotion or to reduce sun exposure in order to prevent skin cancer. Dark pigmented people who use sunscreen are at great disadvantage. Highly melanized skin serves as a sun block which slows the production of vitamin D in the skin of people with dark pigmentation. Applying sunscreen further impedes the production of vitamin D for darkly pigmented people. Regardless of pigmentation, the ability of skin covered with sunscreen to absorb ultraviolet-B rays of the sun is reduced by 90 to 99 percent.

In addition to preventing vitamin D production, you may be harmed by the chemicals in many brands of sunscreen lotion. The Environmental Working Group reported that 15 percent of sunscreen products offer inadequate sunscreen protection and have ingredients that are either hazardous to health or have not been tested for safety. Added to this, a large percentage of sunscreen products do not provide the protection that these products claim to give users. Instead of avoiding the sun dark pigmented people need to get in the sun. There is great need for accurate information about the benefits of sunshine. I advised one of my friends, a dark-skinned man, to make use of the abundant sunlight in his tropical country and I was surprised to hear his response. He replied that sun exposure causes skin cancer so he tries to stay out of the sun. I therefore had the opportunity to advise him about the unique vitamin D needs of dark pigmented people. In order to produce sufficient vitamin D, a dark pigmented person needs to get approximately ten times the sun exposure that a light-skinned person requires.

Get the most from sunlight but ensure your health by taking vitamin D supplements. Vitamin D heals your pain and mellows your mood. It also helps to prevent cancer, high blood pressure, diabetes, arthritis, multiple sclerosis and many more diseases.

Chapter 2

Melanin and Vitamin D: Ironies of Nature

The Melanin Factor

Human skin gets most of its coloring or pigmentation from a chemical compound called melanin. The multitudinous shades of human skin color which range from light shades of ivory to dark browns are a result of differences in the amount of melanin in people's skin. Lightly pigmented skin has less melanin than darkly pigmented skin, which has denser concentrations of melanin.

Skin color evolved as a response to the adaptation of our ancestors to their environment thousands of years ago. Scientists now know that dark skin pigmentation in early humans evolved for two reasons. First, dark skin evolved as a protection mechanism from the intense UVR in equatorial Africa. Second, dark skin color served as a defense mechanism to ensure protection of folate in the body, which is vital for reproductive success.

High concentration of melanin or dark skin pigmentation provided our ancestors with much needed protection from UVR effects that were harmful to health. Through this process, dark pigmented skin with high melanin serves as a natural sun-block or sunscreen thereby offering protection from sunburn and even skin cancer. However, although dark pigmented skin serves as an effective sun-block it also inhibits production of vitamin D in the skin.

Lighter skin color evolved as a response to differing environmental circumstances as early humans migrated from equatorial Africa to high latitude regions with far less intense UVR exposure. The cellular manufacture of vitamin D was needed for survival so people living in Northern latitudes required skin uninhibited by dark pigmentation in order to absorb enough of the less intense sun rays. Under these circumstances light skin pigmentation was needed to increase production of vitamin D.

Dark Skin Pigmentation and Folate

Scientists inform us that the second and less discussed reason for the evolution of dark skin pigmentation was to prevent the destruction of folate in the body from UVR. Folate is necessary for the production of DNA and, consequently, successful repro-duction. Without enough folate an expectant mother will not produce enough DNA to facilitate successful development and growth of a fetus. UVR can destroy folate in the body. Pregnant women with low folate in their blood are at higher risk of having babies born with neural tube birth defects.

Because folate is necessary for DNA production everyone is affected by its impact on health since DNA facilitates a wide range of functions in the body that require cell division. In addition to playing a vital role in embryonic development, DNA cell division processes include producing and replenishing sperm cells in men, skin cells, and hair cells. Since folate is so important to good health, everyone is encouraged to eat foods such as dark green leafy vegetables and whole grains that are rich in folate, and take folate supplements. Women of reproductive age are especially encouraged to consume adequate amounts of folate.

Why Are Dark-Skinned People Predisposed to Vitamin D Deficiency?: The Melanin Factor

Although dark skin evolved to serve vital biological and physiological functions it is not without its ironies. Dark skin helps to protect from harmful UVR and preserve folate necessary for successful reproduction but it also inhibits production of vitamin D from the sun.

God created the universe and fashioned human and other life forms so that life may advantageously exist in its environment. Highly melanized skin or dark skin pigmentation served our ancestors well while they lived in equatorial Africa because high melanin concentration was necessary for protection from the intense rays of the sun.

A dilemma arises when highly melanized skin, which was created to carry out extremely vital biological functions, becomes an impediment to optimum health because of insufficient sun exposure. People with dark skin pigmentation who live in tropical regions and who get sufficient sun exposure are more likely to have good health than people with equally dark skin who live in higher latitudes with limited sunlight. A light pigmented person standing in the sun in an area with relatively low UV radiation will be able to produce enough vitamin D that the body typically requires for one day in about 10 to 15 minutes. In stark contrast, a very dark pigmented person, standing in the same spot will need approximately ten times more sun exposure to produce the same amount of vitamin D. The sunlight needs for dark pigmented people living in northern climates with low UV radiation such as the United States are great and are not being met.

Melanin, Vitamin D and Illness

Dark skin color may protect you but it can also screen the vital sun rays that your body needs to manufacture vitamin D. Statistically, people with dark skin have a higher chance of getting or dying from any of 17 different types of cancers, diabetes, high blood pressure, obesity, heart disease, AIDS, multiple sclerosis, lupus, schizophrenia, and other illnesses. Studies show that blacks suffer greater mortality rates from these diseases.

Black children and adults are in great danger of having low vitamin D in their bodies and of not being able to fight off diseases. In one study, researchers found that during winter, when the sun is weakest, more than ninety-five percent of blacks are deficient in vitamin D. Dark-skinned people who live in cold northern climates with limited sunlight such as the northern USA,

United Kingdom and Canada are more susceptible to being severely deficient in vitamin D. One study that was conducted at Dudley Road Hospital in Birmingham, England found a high prevalence of vitamin D deficiency among Afro-Caribbean and Asians. This underscores the fact that dark-skinned people of different ethnic origins who live in cold, northern climates are highly susceptible to vitamin D deficiency. Dark skin pigmentation blocks ultraviolet-B rays of the sun and further prevents the limited amount of northern sunlight from entering the skin to produce vitamin D. Blacks therefore suffer from more diseases in these regions.

Melanin can work against vitamin D production in dark-skinned individuals even when they live in tropical climates because modern lifestyles have significantly reduced the amount of time people spend outdoors in the sun each day. Blacks living in tropical climates can become significantly deficient in vitamin D if they do not spend about three hours in the sun each day. If you are dark-skinned and you live in a sunlight poor region or cannot find enough time to spend in the sun each day it is imperative that you begin taking vitamin D supplements.

The Function of Vitamin D

What exactly is vitamin D and how does your body get supplied with this substance? Vitamin D is as important to your health as food, shelter, and the air you breathe. It supports all your tissues and organs. Scientists claim that vitamin D is "a near magic pill" or "a miracle working nutrient" because of what it does for your body. However, vitamin D is not really a vitamin. It is a hormone that is produced from cholesterol under your skin. Vitamin D binds to receptors on the membrane outside of cells, and sends signals to the nucleus or brain of each cell. In this way vitamin D causes different changes to take place at the cellular level in the body. Vitamin D acts on more than 2,000 genes in your body. This wonder nutrient is even known to make chemotherapy work better against cancer cells. Researchers tell us that vitamin D eliminates cancer cells by causing these killer cells to change form and become healthy cells. Scientific studies now show that vitamin D is the amazing substance that does all these things when only about twenty years ago it was referred to as the anti-rachitic vitamin because it was known only to prevent rickets in children and bone loss in adults.

The Different Forms of Vitamin D

Vitamin D is also referred to as D3 and D2. Vitamin D3, cholecalciferol, is made naturally in human skin, when sunlight hits the skin. Vitamin D2, or ergocalciferol, is produced in plants and fungi when exposed to sunlight. Many forms of D2 are synthetic. You can take either vitamin D3 or D2 in supplement form, but D2 does not raise your blood vitamin D level as efficiently as D3. It takes more of the D2 form of the vitamin to raise your vitamin D levels to normal, healthy levels.

Despite the fact that D2 is less potent it is the form that is often prescribed by doctors. However, it is better to take the D2 form of vitamin D, than to do without it completely. Vitamin D3 is easily available from reputable companies and many nutritionists and doctors can recommend the more reliable brands. Please see recommendations at the end of the book for reputable vitamin D brands.

Chemical Terms for Vitamin D

Different terms, formulae and numbers are used to identify vitamin D. The active metabolic form of vitamin D is called 1,25-dihydroxyvitamin D (referred to as 1,25-vitamin D). The unactivated form, 25-vitamin D, comes from supplementation or sunlight production under your skin.

Vitamin D Changing Forms Throughout the Body

Vitamin D3 from your skin or from your supplement is transported to your blood. The vitamin is called calcidiol or 25, hydroxyvitamin D in your blood. This is the form that is tested by labs to tell whether or not you are vitamin D deficient. Take note and make sure that this is the vitamin D test that your doctor orders for you. When 25-vitamin D reaches the cells in your body it is converted to the activated form, 1, 25-vitamin D or calcitriol.

Vitamin D Synthesis From the Sun

In order for vitamin D to work as a hormone it must be activated and this process involves a number of steps. Your skin gets exposed to UVB rays from the sun and a type of fat in your skin known as 7-dehydrocholesterol is converted to pre-vitamin D. The next step involves immediate conversion to vitamin D, an active form of vitamin D, in the skin. Vitamin D is further activated in the liver and kidneys where it becomes a powerful hormone which regulates important body functions.

Your skin must be exposed to UVB radiation in order to make the active forms of vitamin D. This puts people with dark skin pigmentation at a disadvantage because highly melanized skin blocks the sun's rays and lowers the amount of vitamin D that can be produced. A dark pigmented person needs to expose eighty-five percent of body surface to the sun during the hours between mid-morning and mid-afternoon for approximately three hours each day in order to get enough vitamin D for optimal health.

Studies inform us that a person with light skin pigmentation will produce 20,000 IU of vitamin D after exposing herself to the sun for 20 minutes, but a dark pigmented individual would need to be exposed to the sun for about 3 hours to make a similar amount of vitamin D. You may be wondering why 20,000 or more International Units (IU) of vitamin D from the sun does not exceed the limit your body can handle. Scientists have found that your body has the capacity to handle large amounts of vitamin D, especially when it comes from the sun. Whenever your body gets all the vitamin D it needs, the sun helps to dispose of excess vitamin D.

How Does Vitamin D Get to Your Cells?

Vitamin D needs to get to your cells to regulate more than two thousand genes in your body and to carry out its health maintaining role. Vitamin D is so vital to your health that the cells in your body carry numerous receptors for this life enhancing substance. Organs of your body have various receiving points for vitamin D. These landing pads are called vitamin D receptors (VDR), and scientists have found that their locations are so numerous that they could be imagined as pins sticking at close intervals all over the body. Vitamin D has different forms but how does the biologically active form get to the cells of your body via these receptors to help fight and control dozens of disease conditions – cancers, heart disease, tuberculosis, swine flu, lupus, diabetes, arthritis and many others?

The Vitamin D Production Process

In the process of getting from your skin to cells of your body, vitamin D binds to proteins and is transported to your liver where it is broken down and further transported to your kidneys and other body organs. In your kidneys and other target organs, vitamin D is changed to a form that is ready to work on the cells in your body. The active form of vitamin D has amazing effects on your body, preventing and controlling diseases and in many cases, saving your life.

Synopsis of the Biochemical Role of Vitamin D

Scientific research continues to show that vitamin D strengthens the immune system so that your body becomes better fortified against diseases. Vitamin D plays a critically important role in keeping you in optimal health. Vitamin D prevents a large number of diseases, including Kaposi Sarcoma of HIV/AIDS and breast, colon, and prostrate cancers. You have probably heard that white blood cells known as T lymphocytes, T cells, play an important role in regulating your immune system. These cells form a second line of defense for your body, helping to fight off dangerous microbes like bacteria and viruses that get inside of your body.

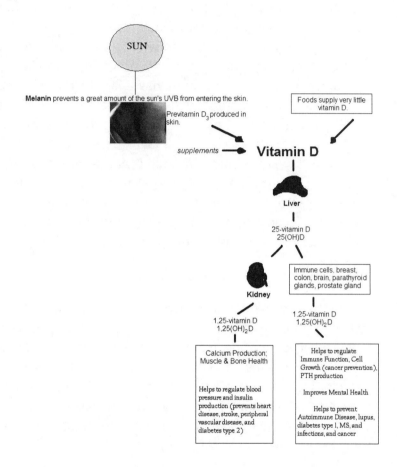

Your immune system is constantly at work, largely powered by these T cells. Vitamin D triggers T cells to destroy bacteria and viruses that invade your body. Vitamin D therefore strengthens T cells, the killer cells of the immune system. Persons with HIV/AIDS or other infections need to keep their vitamin D at an optimal level in order to win the war against dangerous organisms and substances that invade their body. Vitamin D is also a pro-hormone which acts as a powerful antioxidant in reducing lipid peroxidation and preventing diseases. Studies have shown that in the battle against cancer, vitamin D is a far more powerful antioxidant than vitamins C and E. Vitamin D stimulates enzymes that protect your body against oxidation, and by so doing protects you from all kinds of diseases.

The Hormone Balancing Function of Vitamin D

As a steroid hormone, vitamin D forms partnership with other hormones in the body to create balance and regulate the physiology of the human body. This is an extremely important role because hormonal imbalances create disruption of normal body function, resulting in diseases that contribute to further impairment of vital functions of tissues and organs of the body. The possibility exists for vitamin D to be an essential part of treatment plans for diabetes, depression and other illnesses because research has found that vitamin D helps to initiate the production of hormones such as insulin and dopamine. Insulin regulates blood sugar and dopamine modulates mood and memory.

Diabetes is linked to an imbalance of the hormone insulin which regulates blood sugar. Approximately 25 million Americans suffer from this debilitating condition. When your vitamin D levels are inadequate you may end up having too little insulin or be unable to make proper use of insulin thereby predisposing you to diabetes. Consequently, glucose accumulates in your blood causing an abnormal increase in your blood sugar level. Vitamin D helps to stimulate the body to make proper use of insulin that is produced in the body.

Vitamin D deficiency could be one of the underlying reasons why so many black people are diabetic. Statistics from the United States Centers for Disease Control and Prevention show that blacks suffer higher rates of diabetes than whites, and scientific studies inform us that more than 95 percent of blacks have insufficient vitamin D in their blood. Dark skin pigmentation prevents production of vitamin D from the sun so dark-skinned people are usually lower in vitamin D and this leads to insufficient insulin to remove sugar from the blood. Therefore many more dark pigmented persons are likely to become diabetic. Vitamin D has been shown to help prevent and control both type 1 and type 2 diabetes. One study reported on in a 2010 issue of the *Australian Medical Journal* found that vitamin D supplementation positively affects the insulin status of vitamin D-deficient women. After supplementation with vitamin D, the women showed improved insulin sensitivity.

Mental illness is another condition that is often linked to hormonal imbalance. Fifty million Americans are mentally ill. Vitamin D deficiency is linked to depression, chronic fatigue and other brain ailments. According to the *FASEB Journal,* there is ample biological evidence to show that vitamin D plays an important role in brain development and function. *The Vitamin D Council* reports that epidemiological evidence shows that reduced sun-exposure, and low blood vitamin D may cause or worsen mental illness. *The Vitamin D Council* also informs us that studies show that mental illness improves when sufficient vitamin D is given to patients. Additionally, vitamin D deficiency contributes to people becoming more depressed during the winter months and serious deficiency of this vitamin is said to be responsible for many cases of clinical depression and schizophrenia.

Vitamin D affects dopamine, a brain hormone. When your body is deficient in vitamin D, there may be insufficient pro-duction of the hormone dopamine, so you are likely to become depressed, unable to concentrate, exhausted or experience chronic fatigue. Dopamine is a neurotransmitter that regulates mood and memory. Studies show that deficiency of vitamin D may also lead to Attention Deficit Hyperactive Disorder (ADD/HD) in children. Statistics show that disproportionate numbers of black children are placed in Special Education classes and are being treated for hyperactive disorder. It is likely that vitamin D deficiency contributes to ADD/HD in black children because researchers at Harvard Medical School, the University of

Colorado-Denver, and Massachusetts General Hospital found that 92 percent of black children are deficient in vitamin D.

Dietary Sources of Vitamin D May Be Insufficient

Foods do not supply enough vitamin D to maintain your health and multivitamins will not give you an adequate amount either. Furthermore, the vitamin D content in packaged foods and multivitamins is based on the U.S. recommended daily allowance (RDA) for nutrients. The RDA for vitamin D is 600 IU, which is a small fraction of the amount that you need to maintain optimum health. Milk that is sold in the United States, Canada, and some European countries is fortified with vitamin D. Many brands of orange juice, margarine, and cereals also contain vitamin D, but you should not depend on these sources to supply the amount of vitamin D that your body requires. These foods and drinks contain much less vitamin D than your body needs and one study found that some foods contain even lesser amounts than the food labels show. Think for a minute of how inadequate your food supply can be: in order to get an amount of vitamin D equal to the measure you would get from 3 hours of sun exposure, you would need to drink about 400 glasses of milk! And, in order to get 1,000 IU of vitamin D per day (less than the amount your body is likely to need) you would have to consume ten eight-ounce glasses of milk each day.

Although the crucial link between chronic vitamin D deficiency in blacks and the alarmingly high rates of diseases they suffer has recently been established, many people are still unaware of this potentially life-saving information. Thus, notwithstanding the relatively inexpensive and simple way to meet the unique vitamin D needs of darkly pigmented people, rates of chronic diseases related to vitamin D deficiency continue to skyrocket among blacks. The following chapter delves further into examining the problem of vitamin D deficiency among blacks by contrasting the rates of chronic diseases among darkly pigmented people with lightly pigmented people.

Chapter 3

Disproportionate Disease and Mortality Rates Among Blacks

Vitamin D deficiency is at epidemic proportions in the United States and it is worse among blacks. A national sample of almost 19,000 people, taken over a 16-year period, from 1988 to 2004, shows that the proportion of Americans with healthy vitamin D levels fell from 45 percent to 23 percent. During this same period, the number of blacks with adequate vitamin D in their blood plummeted from 12 percent to an alarming level of 3 percent. Indeed, this is cause for great concern because vitamin D is rightly called the "miracle nutrient," responsible for a host of important biological functions in the body, and a major contributor to a well-functioning immune system and good health. Vitamin D improves antibacterial, antiviral and anti-parasitic functioning of the immune system and people with low vitamin D levels in their blood are more likely to die from cancer, heart disease, stroke, and many other diseases.

Recent scientific research points to strong evidence that vitamin D deficiency causes high blood pressure, heart disease, strokes, diabetes, asthma, at least seventeen types of cancer, chronic pain, and dozens of other diseases. Further, the United States Centers for Disease Control and Prevention informs us that blacks suffer the highest disease and mortality rates. There is strong evidence that the health of many blacks is being seriously compromised because they have critically low vitamin D in their bodies. However, the conventional health care system is doing an unsatisfactory job of educating people with dark skin pigmentation about their vitamin D deficiency and resulting vulnerability. A study reported on in the November 2010 issue of the *Journal of the American Medical Association* suggests that addressing the vitamin D needs of African Americans may be the single most important public health measure that can be undertaken, due to the widespread vitamin D deficiency in the black population and the health benefits that can be derived from adequate vitamin D levels.

Whether you live in cold Alaska, hot Atlanta or sun-drenched Florida you may become deficient in vitamin D. In fact, vitamin D deficiency is common all over the world. People who live in the Caribbean, Africa, and India also show high rates of vitamin D deficiency and many suffer from diseases that are related to vitamin D deficiency. Leading vitamin D researcher, Dr. Michael Holick reports that 50 to 80 percent of adults, including 90 percent of medical doctors living in various parts of India, and more than 50 percent of children living in New Delhi, the capital city of India, had low vitamin D blood levels.

Physicians believe it is inflammation in the body that causes most of the chronic diseases in humans, and researchers confirm that insufficient vitamin D is a major contributor to these diseases. Cancer, diabetes, heart disease, lupus and schizophrenia are some of the most disabling and deadly diseases that may result from inflammation in the body. Black people suffer the most from these chronic inflammatory diseases since pigmentation in darker skin blocks the necessary ultraviolet rays of the sun. According to current research, if you are black and you have not been taking at least 5,000 International Units of vitamin D per day, you may get sick or become sicker.

When you get an infection, ranging from a simple cold to cancer, your immune system kicks in to help your body recover. However, if your immune system is not performing properly, you become chronically ill. Scientists have recently found out that most cells of your immune system including T cells and others called antigen presenting cells and macrophages have vitamin D receptors. These receptors are there for the extremely important purpose of receiving vitamin D. Strong evidence shows that vitamin D has a number of important effects on your immune system. If you are dark-skinned there is a good chance that you do not have enough vitamin D in your body to enhance your innate immunity and prevent diseases.

Interestingly, many physicians have been stumbling on vitamin D deficiency among dark-skinned people but have probably given no serious thought to what they found. One of my friends who resided in Britain for many years told me about discussions she had with doctors there. Doctors she visited wondered why dark-skinned Africans and Afro-Caribbeans living in Britain have such high rates of arthritis and asthma. I share similar concerns and often discuss this with family members and friends.

As I walk on the streets of New York City, I see a disproportionate number of dark-skinned people using ambulatory aids such as walking sticks and walkers. Whether they are rich or poor, educated or uneducated, or living in tropical or temperate geographical zones, when taken as a group, blacks have the highest rates of chronic diseases and these rates are skyrocketing. Researchers point to a common thread as a major contributing factor to the high rates of chronic disease among blacks – highly melanized skin that causes dark-skinned people to be deficient in vitamin D.

The Myth of Faulty Lifestyle Practices Among Blacks

You have probably heard a lot about high rates of poverty and illiteracy among blacks and how these social maladies predispose blacks to adopting unhealthy lifestyle practices that destroy their health. Notwithstanding these arguments, studies have shown that socioeconomic status and lifestyle practices do not explain the disproportionate disease burden carried by blacks. In one such study researchers at Harvard University examined diet, lifestyle, and medical risks of African American men from diverse socioeconomic backgrounds. After adjusting for all these variables they found that these black men, regardless of socioeconomic background, had a 32 percent higher risk of getting cancer and an incredible 90 percent higher risk of dying from cancer.

Report on One New York City Neighborhood

To further unravel the myth of faulty lifestyle behaviors being the main cause of the disparate rates of disease among blacks, let us examine a predominantly black community in New York City and compare it with neighboring communities that are predominantly white. According to a New York City Community Health Profile released by the New York City Department of Health, the poverty level in the East Flatbush Community in Brooklyn, New York, is similar to other communities in the city. This community which is 79.2 percent black, has a poverty level of 21 percent, making it wealthier than the Borough of Brooklyn, which has a poverty level of 25 percent, and equal to New York City which also has a 21 percent poverty level. Note that this community probably has the largest number of blacks in the city because 79 percent of East Flatbush is black, while Brooklyn and New York City have 34 percent and 24 percent blacks, respectively.

A *New York Times* report on neighborhoods informs us that this East Flatbush community, largely made up of Afro-Caribbean and African Americans, has a median income of $46,878. The two communities which come closest to the median income in East Flatbush are predominantly white communities (with an average of 75 percent of residents being white). *The New York Times* informs that these two communities have median incomes of $42,314 and $40,412 while the median income for East Flatbush is $46,878. You may also take note that the median income in the U.S. during the same period was reported to be $42,000. Formal education attainment in East Flatbush is also above New York City's average. Forty-two percent of residents over the age of twenty-five have completed some college education whereas 20 percent of New York City residents have some college education. In addition, more East Flatbush residents than New York City residents completed high school when compared to high school completion rates for the city in general. The New York City Community Health Profile also reports that a high percentage of East Flatbush residents use condoms during sex and engage in less binge drinking than neighboring communities.

Given these facts we have to question why it is that the community of East Flatbush has an alarmingly high rate of 70 HIV/AIDS cases per 100,000 residents, while Brooklyn has 50 per 100,000 and New York City has 55 per 100,000. It is worth considering that chronic vitamin D deficiency could be a major contributing factor to the disproportionately high rates of HIV/AIDS cases among residents in this East Flatbush community. The following chapter examines in further detail the disproportionate illness rates among dark pigmented people and the relationship of this phenomenon to vitamin D deficiency among dark-skinned people.

Chapter 4

Vitamin D's Role in Preventing and Controlling Major Diseases:
Immune Disorders

HIV/AIDS in Blacks and Whites – U.S. Statistics

The number of HIV/AIDS cases among blacks has been at epidemic levels for some time. AIDS continues to be the leading killer of young African Americans between 25 and 44 years, with more blacks dying from AIDS than from homicide, drugs and alcohol, cancer and heart disease combined. African Americans comprise 12 percent of the U.S. population but more than 40 percent of new HIV/AIDS cases. Young black women make up the greatest percentage of new AIDS cases. *The Balm in Gilead*, an organization that mounts an HIV/AIDS informational campaign through black churches, has been doing a monumental job that can be greatly enhanced with information from recent studies about vitamin D's role in helping to reduce disease progression in HIV/AIDS.

People with HIV may help prevent opportunistic diseases, prevent AIDS and lead healthier lives when they have an adequate amount of vitamin D in their blood. A recent study conducted by researchers at Harvard University found that low vitamin D status is significantly associated with progression of HIV-related diseases to more dangerous stages. Scientists point to vitamin D deficiency as a major cause of the greater number of AIDS cases in the

African American population. Blacks are known to be critically deficient in vitamin D so they may have more difficulty fighting opportunistic diseases that are caused by the HIV virus. They therefore get sicker and die faster from HIV/AIDS.

HIV/AIDS in Blacks and Whites

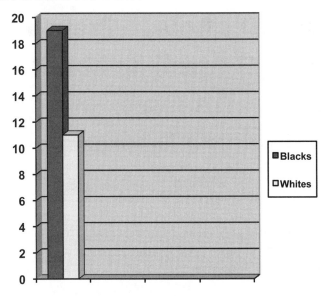

Estimated number of AIDS cases in the United States in 2007
Blacks: 18, 500 HIV/AIDS cases   Whites: 11, 000 HIV/AIDS cases

Vitamin D deficiency weakens the immune system and a weakened immune system cannot effectively fight off opportunistic infections brought on by HIV. The immune system has cells that are specially equipped to engulf and kill viral-infected cells, tumor cells and bacteria. T-cells in the immune system are some of these specialized bodies, called lymphocytes. HIV causes gradual depletion of T-cells but vitamin D can work in conjunction with daily consumption of nourishing meals and appropriate medical treatment to improve the quality of life of persons living with HIV. Vitamin D is a potent anti-inflammatory substance that helps the proper functioning of T-cells. Vitamin D supplements may also help to reduce HIV infection mortality rates in children.

One study reported on in a 2009 issue of the *Journal of Infectious Diseases* found that children born to HIV-infected mothers with low vitamin D levels have a 61 percent risk of dying very early.

African Americans make up 12 percent of the United States population but carry approximately 45 percent of the HIV/AIDS infection burden. AIDS-related diagnoses and deaths peaked in the 1990s but have been constant since then. The chart above is based on statistics from the United States Centers for Disease Control and Prevention and represents AIDS cases in the 50 contiguous states.

Lupus and Multiple Sclerosis

In an attempt to protect itself from disease-causing agents, the body often attacks itself and damages its own cells and tissues. This inappropriate immune-mediated attack on body tissues results in an autoimmune disease. Systemic lupus erythematosus (lupus), and multiple sclerosis (MS) are two of these autoimmune diseases from which blacks suffer disproportionately. An immune system that works properly will not attack cells of its fellow tissues. A healthy immune system has T cells that are properly geared to defend the body from invading microbes such as viruses and bacteria. Optimal vitamin D levels make T cells more efficient at fighting off disease causing microorganisms. Vitamin D supplementation has been found to be useful in preventing the body from destroying its own cells and in lessening the severity of pre-existing autoimmune disease.

Young Black Women Suffer Disproportionately from Lupus

Lupus is an autoimmune disorder that affects virtually any organ of the body. Some of the symptoms of lupus are painful swollen joints, puffy eyes, swollen feet, legs and hands, extreme tiredness, headaches, fever, anemia, abnormal blood clotting, painful chest and difficult breathing, sensitivity to sunlight, and ulcers around the mouth and nose.

Unfortunately, lupus appears to be a mystery disease to medical personnel. The U.S. Centers for Disease Control and Prevention reports that there is no known cause for lupus. This disease is very common in African American females and is often found in people of Asian origin. Many people of Asian origin also have dark skin pigmentation so they may be at risk for lupus because of high concentrations of melanin in their skin. A study published in the April 2008 issue of the *Scandinavian Journal of Immunology* found that blood tests from 123 new systemic lupus erythematosus (SLE) patients showed that their vitamin D levels were much lower than in healthy individuals. The study also found that in this group, African American patients had lower vitamin D levels than Caucasians. Further, patients with the lowest levels of vitamin D had more severe cases of the disease.

Lupus in Black Women and White Women

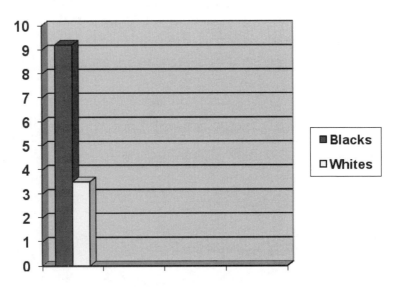

Lupus per 100,000 of population (Source: CDC 2007)
Black Women: 9   White Women: 3.5

Lupus in Black Men and White Men

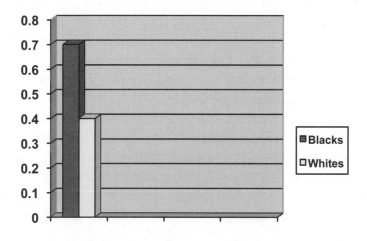

Lupus per 100,000 of population   (Source: CDC 2007)
Black Men: 0.7   White Men: 0.4

Multiple Sclerosis Is More Aggressive in Blacks

Multiple Sclerosis (MS) has been found to run a more aggressive course in blacks. MS is an autoimmune disease in which the immune system attacks the central nervous system and causes destruction of the myelin sheath that covers the nerves. MS is reported to be the most common neurological disorder in Western countries. It causes nervous disability and usually takes a progressive course, giving patients little hope for recovery. It is believed that family members of MS patients are at risk of getting MS because of their genetic predisposition but vitamin D can help to prevent and control this disease. A study reported on in a 2009 issue of *Neurology Reviews* found that increasing evidence shows a link between vitamin D deficiency and multiple sclerosis. Researchers have found that high doses of vitamin D, taken in supplement form, are safe and effective in reducing relapse in patients with MS. Another recent study conducted in Australia also found that inadequate sun exposure and low vitamin D are risk factors for multiple sclerosis.

Vitamin D receptors in the nervous system receive and distribute vitamin D, and vitamin D maintains the growth of myelin around nerve cells. Vitamin D deficiency in MS patients can worsen because patients may find it difficult to spend time outdoors where they are exposed to sunlight. In addition, when MS sufferers reside in regions above 35 degrees latitude, they get no vitamin D from sunlight for many months of the year. It is therefore necessary for these MS sufferers to take optimal dosages of vitamin D.

Geographical location influences the incidence and severity of multiple sclerosis. Researchers mapped the course and distribution of MS cases and found that it was most prevalent in the northern United States, Canada and northern parts of Europe where there is very limited sunshine. Scientists have come to the conclusion that vitamin D plays an important role in preventing and controlling MS. Whenever blacks get this disease, they are at greater risk of dying because MS is more aggressive and disabling in blacks. Dark-skinned people living in the northern region of the United States are in greater danger because this region has shorter periods of sunlight and produces less vitamin D. While it may not be convenient for MS sufferers to correct their vitamin D deficiency through sun-exposure, supplements can be taken to help address the problem.

Asthma

The United States Centers for Disease Control and Prevention reports that more blacks visit physicians' offices and hospital out-patient centers for cases of asthma attacks than whites. Blacks also die from asthma in greater numbers. The *Respiratory Health Association of Metropolitan Chicago* reports that Chicago is an epicenter for asthma, leading the United States in asthma deaths, visits to emergency rooms, and hospitalizations from asthma. The *Missouri Department of Health and Senior Services* informs us that African Americans make up 12 percent of Missouri's population but account for more than 40 percent of emergency room visits due to asthma, nearly five times more than whites.

Numerous studies have linked vitamin D deficiency to asthma. One such study conducted by researchers from Harvard

Medical School and published in the *Journal of Allergy and Clinical Immunology* reports that relatively low vitamin D levels make children more susceptible to severe asthma attacks. For the purposes of this study, researchers defined blood levels below 30 ng/ml as vitamin D insufficiency. The sample size for the study comprised 1,024 children. Thirty-five percent of the children were found to be vitamin D deficient with the African American children in the study having the lowest vitamin D levels and white children having the highest levels. Over the four-year period of the study, researchers found that the children with the lowest vitamin D levels had increased risk of having severe asthma attacks as well as higher odds of hospitalization or emergency room visits. Daily supplementation with vitamin D could save thousands of people from asthma attacks and deaths from these attacks.

Black Athletes, Asthma and Vitamin D Deficiency

Researchers have found that exercise-induced asthma is very common in athletes. Exercise-induced bronchospasm or asthma is five times more common in athletes than in the general population. In one study involving 107 varsity athletes from Ohio, almost 50 percent of the athletes had exercise induced asthma, with most having no history of asthma attacks prior to becoming athletes.

Black athletes have suffered many incidents of asthma attacks while they engage in competitive sports. In late summer 2009, a Chicago Bulls player developed exercise-induced asthma and a Chicago high school football player collapsed on the field and died after suffering an asthma attack. Another black athlete, a 16 year-old varsity football player, died in Cincinnati, Ohio, shortly after practice in August 2010. Yet another black athlete, a basketball player on the United States men's basketball team, thought that the occasional fatigue and shortness of breath from which he suffered were due to poor physical conditioning. He later found out that he had asthma. In September 2010, a seventeen-year-old high school athlete suffered an asthma attack after scoring a touchdown in Oregon. These are but a few of the numerous cases involving black athletes suffering asthma attacks, sometimes fatally.

Researchers recommend that athletes keep their vitamin D, calcium, and magnesium levels optimized in order to help prevent inflammation and bronchospasm which are associated with asthma. Vitamin D helps to inhibit the onset of asthma while calcium and magnesium help to prevent the bronchi or air tubes from going into spasm. Athletes sweat heavily during athletic activities and profuse sweating during such intense physical activities excretes magnesium. This often leads to depletion of magnesium stores in the body. Asthmatic attacks, heart attacks,

Asthma in Blacks and Whites

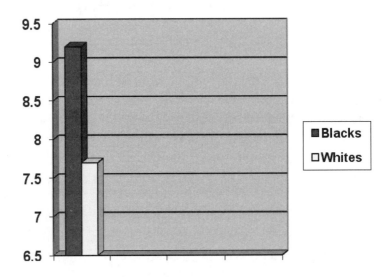

Asthma Death Rate per 100,000 of population (Source: CDC 2007)
Blacks: 9.2   Whites 7.9

and sudden cardiac deaths are very often caused from vitamin D, magnesium, and calcium deficiency. Chapter 5 of this book suggests the amounts of calcium and magnesium that should be consumed on a daily basis. Chapter 10 gives recommendations for vitamin D dosages.

Vitamin D Improves Athletic Performance

Athletes who are deficient in vitamin D are susceptible not only to asthma, but to many other conditions that may afflict them. These conditions include musculoskeletal injuries and poor balance. Studies have shown a positive association between adequate vitamin D levels and peak athletic performance. In keeping with the beneficial effects of UVB irradiance on physical performance, studies have shown that peak athletic performance is associated with the late summer months and a reduction in performance is seen in early autumn when vitamin D levels begin to decline as a result of reduced UVB exposure.

Dark-skinned athletes, because of high melanin concentration which blocks sunlight from entering their skin, are especially vulnerable to the diseases associated with vitamin D deficiency which commonly afflict athletes. Even dark-skinned athletes who live in tropical zones are at risk of vitamin D deficiency if they train indoors. Athletes who live in sunlight rich regions and who train outdoors in such environments often demonstrate impressive athletic performance.

It is easy to appreciate the effects of sunlight and vitamin D on athletic performance when one looks at the usual stellar performance of many African athletes in the annual New York City Marathon. In 2010, two long distance runners from Africa, Edna Kiplagat of Kenya and Gebre Gebremariam of Ethiopia, won the women's and men's titles, respectively. They outperformed 42,000 other runners from all over the world who participated in the New York City Marathon in 2010. We now know that adequate vitamin D levels obtained from UVB irradiance plays an important role in enhancing the endurance and strength of stellar athletes such as those from Africa and the Caribbean.

Some researchers have highlighted the impressive number of world records set during the 1968 summer Olympics in Mexico City as further evidence that vitamin D improves athletic performance. Americans performed exceptionally well that year, winning the majority of the gold medals in outdoor sports, with long jumper Bob Beamon adding 21 inches to the World Record for long jump and setting a new record of 29 feet. Russians also performed well as they won most of the gold medals for indoor sports. Researchers believe that the intense UVB irradiation to which the athletes were exposed during the 1968 summer Olympics in Mexico City rapidly increased their vitamin D levels, thus resulting in the exceptional performances and new world records that were set that summer.

Rheumatoid Arthritis

Rheumatoid arthritis is an inflammatory disease in which arthritis develops in the joints and sometimes the eyes and lungs. Symptoms include numbness or tingling in joints of the fingers and toes, stiffness of the joints for extended period of time, joint deformities in hands and feet, low grade fever, and loss of appetite. These symptoms may appear singly or be combined. This disease can be quite severe, leading to damaged joints, deformed spine, heart disease, lung dysfunction and damage of nerves and blood vessels. Over the counter arthritis medication is often used in an effort to reduce the inflammation of the joints but these may cause many serious side effects. Rheumatoid arthritis is more common in people of color and the disease also runs a more aggressive course in blacks. It is more common in women than men and generally affects the smaller joints such as those of the hands and feet – knuckles, wrists, ankles and toes.

The October 2010 edition of the *Journal of Rheumatology* reports on a study involving a population of 850 mostly elderly men with rheumatoid arthritis. The researchers found that there is a link between vitamin D deficiency and the prevalence and severity of rheumatoid arthritis. Researchers have found that adequate supplementation with vitamin D can reduce inflammation and improve symptoms. Osteoarthritis, which should not be confused with rheumatoid arthritis, is a more common form of arthritis that results from "wear-and-tear" of the joints of the body. This form of arthritis usually occurs in elderly people and typically affects the larger weight-bearing joints of the body, knees, hips, areas generally not affected by rheumatoid arthritis.

Arthritis in Blacks and Whites

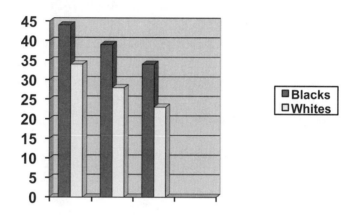

Activity Limitation: Blacks 44 percent, Whites 34 percent   (Source: CDC 2007)
Work Limitation: Blacks 39 percent, Whites 28 percent
Severe Joint Pain: Blacks 34 percent, Whites 23 percent

Uterine Fibroids in Women

A recent finding confirms that vitamin D may regulate estrogen and retard the growth of fibroids in the uterus. A study conducted by researchers at *Meharry Medical College*, the largest private historically black academic health center in the United States, shows that vitamin D may help to slow the growth of fibroids of the uterus. The study, which was reported on in the August 2010 issue of *Fertility and Sterility,* found that vitamin D disrupts the production of enzymes in human fibroid cells. Vitamin D affects the production of the enzyme catechol-O-methyltransferase and this may inhibit the growth of human uterine fibroid cells by 47 percent. Catechol-O-methyltransferase helps to control estrogen production. This enzyme, therefore, prevents estrogen-induced growths such as fibroids of the uterus.

Uterine fibroids occur 3-5 times more often in black women than in white women and vitamin D deficiency may be a trigger for the growth of these abnormal tissues in the uterus. Black women may derive significant health benefit by taking vitamin D supplements because they experience higher incidence of uterine fibroids and suffer greater deficiencies of vitamin D. Findings from the *Meharry Medical College* study bring hope for women because uterine fibroids can cause profuse menstrual bleeding and pelvic pain. Fibroids of the uterus are noncancerous tumors that usually cause no symptoms and may not require treatment. However, these tumors may also cause infertility and pregnancy complications. Fibroid tumors affect as many as 77 percent of women in the United States.

Chapter 5

Vitamin D and Its Cofactors Help Prevent Heart Disease, Diabetes, and Obesity

Hypertension or high blood pressure is an epidemic among African Americans. A study reported on in a 2009 issue of the *Journal of Thrombosis and Haemostasis* found a 60 percent increased risk of heart and blood vessel disease among blacks, when compared to whites. One in 3 African American women suffers from high blood pressure and if the current trend continues, one half of all African Americans will die from stroke or heart disease. Uncontrolled high blood pressure can cause heart disease, the rupture of an artery, and bleeding within the brain and other tissues. Having high blood pressure puts you at increased risk of sudden death from a heart attack.

Numerous studies have shown that vitamin D can help to lower the incidence of high blood pressure. While carrying out its metabolic functions throughout the body vitamin D forms products that have anticoagulant properties which help to prevent hyper coagulation or thickening of the blood. Vitamin D therefore controls blood pressure, prevents blood clots, reduces the incidence of stroke and minimizes one's risk for heart disease. One study involving a group of over 12, 000 people examined the effects of vitamin D on high blood pressure. The study found a positive correlation between low vitamin D levels and high blood pressure. Elderly persons with low vitamin D levels were found to be more susceptible to getting high blood pressure. The study also found that vitamin D affects high blood pressure more significantly in elderly persons. In this study, when vitamin D levels were increased from 20 to 100 nmol/L, blood pressure decreased by 1.8 mmhg in people below the age of 50. A similar increase in vitamin D levels caused blood pressure to be lowered by 4.6 mmhg in persons above the age of 50. The study points out that even a small reduction in high blood pressure can result in significantly lower rates of heart disease.

Many studies confirm that insufficient vitamin D in the blood can lead to heart disease. One large scale study involving 15, 000 participants was carried out by researchers at the University of Rochester. The study examined the risk of death from cardiovascular disease for people who had low vitamin D levels. The researchers found that those with low vitamin D levels had a 40 percent higher chance of dying from heart disease. They also found that patients had insufficient vitamin D levels prior to developing cardio-vascular related conditions such as high blood pressure. Some researchers believe that it may be helpful to have vitamin D supplementation trials on blacks, who bear a greater burden for heart disease.

Vitamin D deficiency during the early years may lay the foundation for development of high blood pressure later in life. Some researchers believe that vitamin D deficiency during the early years and beyond might have an adverse effect on the small blood vessels in the body. Early and extended vitamin D deficiency might be a contributing factor to the high rates of high blood pressure among African Americans.

Heart Disease in Young Black Adults

Heart disease is more common in young African Americans than their white counterparts. African Americans between the ages of 35 and 44 years have twice as much heart disease as whites. Blacks also suffer heart attacks at younger ages than whites. Abnormal heart functioning and/or hypertension during the twenties, thirties and forties, are oftentimes predictive of heart failure later in life.

Researchers at Emory University in Atlanta, Georgia, carried out a recent vitamin D supplementation study of black teens in the United States. These researchers compared an experimental high dosage group with a group that received the regular Required Daily Allowance (RDA) which was 400 International Units (IU) at the time of the study. The experimental high dosage group received 2,000 IU of vitamin D each day. Significant differences were seen between the group that received 2,000 IU of vitamin D daily, and the group that got 400 IU (RDA), per day. At the end of the 16 week study, the black teens who received the higher dosage of 2,000 IU of vitamin D experienced significant improvement in the rate of flow of oxygenated blood throughout the arteries and were in better health than those who received the lower dosage of 400 IU. The teens who received 400 IU per day, showed worsened central arterial stiffness.

Heart Attacks During Winter

People with vitamin D deficiency tend to get sick during the winter months or shortly after winter when the vitamin D-producing UVB rays from the sun are less intense and in some cases non-existent. *The Journal of Thrombosis and Haemostasis* reports that a cohort study comprising 40,000 women from the southern Swedish population shows that diseases of the blood vessels and heart increase by about 50 percent during winter. Here's an example of a case involving a dark-skinned heart attack victim who suffered heart attacks during the winter months with the last one being fatal.

It was towards the end of winter when Louise got a very frightening call about her sister who lived in England. Her nephew's voice on the other end of the line said, "Auntie, I'm sorry to tell you this, but mom had a heart attack." On hearing this Louise almost had a heart attack also. Louise called an airline, booked her passage from New York and headed off to England. Fortunately the heart attack was not fatal so she was able to spend some time with her ailing sister before returning home.

A few years later Louise received another call about her sister. She had suffered a second heart attack. This second attack also occurred shortly after winter. Her sister's vitamin D levels appeared to have again gotten depleted during the winter months in the cold northern climate in England. A few years later, a third heart attack claimed the life of Louise's sister. Her sister did not take any vitamin D supplements.

Louise's sister fits the profile of someone who is susceptible to high blood pressure, strokes and heart attacks — dark-skinned and living in a high latitude region with poor sun exposure. If current statistical data hold true, 50 percent of black women living in the United States, will die from a heart attack or stroke. Needless to say, dark pigmented people living in other sunlight poor northern regions such as Canada or Europe also face great risk of dying from heart attacks or strokes. However, with proper diet and vitamin D supplementation these statistics can be changed to reflect more positive outcomes.

Sugar Adversely Affects Your Blood Pressure

High blood pressure is a major contributing factor to cardiovascular disease and other major chronic illnesses. Do you wonder why your blood pressure is abnormally high and will not decrease, or why your cholesterol is high? Numerous studies have shown that sugar raises uric acid levels in your body which leads to a number of health complications including high blood pressure, elevated low density lipoprotein, LDL (bad cholesterol), insulin resistance, diabetes, obesity and even pre-eclampsia in pregnant women. Sucrose or ordinary table sugar is formed from two simple sugars – glucose and fructose. When sugar enters your body, the fructose component is metabolized and produces waste products that are bad for your health. Uric acid is one of the waste products formed from fructose. Uric acid drives up your blood pressure by inhibiting nitric oxide in your blood vessels. Nitric oxide helps your blood vessels maintain their elasticity so that your blood flows at a healthy pressure. When you avoid using sugars such as high fructose corn syrup, you help to normalize your blood pressure. High fructose corn syrup is often found in sodas and many processed foods available today. It is a healthy habit to read food labels carefully and limit the use of all types of sugar and foods containing sugar.

When you take vitamin D supplements and avoid excessive sugar in your diet, you are helping to control high blood pressure while preventing other diseases. This is much like killing many birds with one stone. Some experts believe that even with a blood pressure reading that is accepted as normal, but on the high end of normal, your chance of developing cancer is raised to 68 percent, your chance of early death from any cause increases by 46 percent, and the probability of developing cardiovascular disease increases by 33 percent. Vitamin D is like a magic bullet hitting many health robbers with one shot.

Get to the Root of What Causes Your High Blood Pressure

High blood pressure is triggered by numerous underlying causes which place undue stress on your body organs. New studies show that vitamin D helps to prevent high blood pressure because it assists with healthy functioning of the endothelial cells of blood vessels. These are thin cells that line your blood vessels. These cells are thin enough to allow nutrients from your food and other substances, beneficial or toxic, to get across to your blood or be excreted from your blood. Your blood transports materials to and from your body cells and organs of your body. Waste products of metabolism get filtered from body organs into the blood stream and these wastes get moved along to excretory organs such as your kidneys and skin.

Vitamin D can help to combat silent but dangerous bio-chemical activities in your body that contribute to hypertension. Environmental health educator Dr Sherry Rogers, points out that viruses and bacteria may cause damage to your blood vessels and cells of your body which may contribute to high blood pressure. Bacteria and viruses may enter your body and cause no symptoms for years, but silently damage the walls of your blood vessels. In the meantime you may be eating foods that contain high percentages of trans fats. These include junk foods that cause the lining of your blood vessels to get weaker. The bugs in your body continually chew on your weakening blood vessel lining, setting up infections in your arteries. Naked electrons called free radicals bombard your cells and tissues on a constant basis. You get these free radicals from more than 60, 000 disease causing chemicals in your food, water, and the air you breathe. You need adequate vitamin D and other antioxidant foods to neutralize and destroy free radicals that can cause your blood pressure to be stubbornly high. Vitamin D along with foods that nourish, detoxify and bolster your immune system can help to prevent and control high blood pressure.

Vitamin D is a powerful antioxidant that can remove toxins from your body, prevent and heal damaged blood vessels, and regulate your circulatory system so that your blood flows at a healthy pressure to all of your body organs. Unfortunately, blacks do not make enough vitamin D so they have higher rates of high blood pressure, stroke and heart disease.

You Need to Have Enough Blood Calcium, Magnesium, and Vitamin K2

Magnesium, calcium, and Vitamin K2 are cofactors of vitamin D. Together with vitamin D, they work to prevent or reverse high blood pressure and to control heart disease. It is therefore very important that your diet include foods and supplements that contain magnesium, calcium, and vitamin K2, because these nutrients work together with vitamin D to maintain your health. Remember that these nutrients work synergetically as nature intended. They are not meant to be taken in isolation.

The Importance of Magnesium

Magnesium is used in more than 300 enzyme related biochemical reactions in your body and is needed in abundance to work with calcium to maintain healthy contraction and relaxation of your heart muscle and healthy operation of blood vessels. In fact, magnesium deficiency can trigger a large number of illnesses. Lower levels of magnesium in the blood can lead to migraine headaches, anxiety, depression, diabetes, high blood pressure and other illnesses. Experts advise that you take about 400 to 700 mg of magnesium each day because magnesium has been signifycantly depleted in soils that grow our food. Additional deficiencies are created in fruit and vegetable crops because plant fertilizers with excess amounts of potassium and phosphorus reduce the ability of plants to take up magnesium from the soil. In addition to nutrient deficient soil and low uptake by plants, food processing and faulty meal preparation methods help to remove magnesium from foods. High blood pressure medication, insulin abnormalities, advancing age, and mental stress also cause magnesium levels to be reduced in the body. Magnesium deficiency is said to be one of the causes of the many degenerative diseases that we have not been able to control.

Low magnesium is also linked to heart disease and death from heart disease. As many as 80 percent of Americans may be deficient in magnesium. The United States Centers for Disease Control and Prevention reports that 250,000 people die from sudden cardiac arrest each year. Death from cardiac arrest, abrupt loss of heartbeat or heart function, may or may not involve any history of heart disease. One study published in a 2010 issue of The *American Journal of Clinical Nutrition* found that sudden death from cardiac arrest was much lower in people with the highest levels of magnesium in their blood. The study examined magnesium intake in 88,375 women and found that there was a 40 percent reduced chance of suffering sudden cardiac death when blood magnesium level was high. Magnesium is so vital to proper heart functioning that it is often administered intravenously during cases of cardiac arrest. If you choose to take a magnesium supplement it is important that it is balanced with calcium and vitamin D as all these nutrients are meant to work together for optimum health.

Calcium Helps Prevent High Blood Pressure

High blood pressure and abnormal contraction of heart muscles have been associated with insufficient calcium levels. Excellent dietary sources of calcium include dark green leafy vegetables, peas, beans and other vegetables, and sardines. Ade-

Daily Calcium Requirements	
Age	Calcium
1-3 years	700 mg/day
4-8 years	1,000 mg/day
9-18 years	1,300 mg/day
19-50 years	1,000 mg/day
51 years and older	1,200 mg/day
Postmenopausal Women	1,500 mg/day
Pregnant and Breastfeeding Women	1,300 mg/day

Recommended daily calcium needs for different age groups
Source: National Institutes of Health

High Blood Pressure in Black Women and White Women

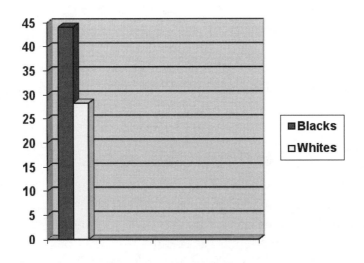

High Blood Pressure per 100,000 of population (Source: CDC 2007)
Black Women: 44   White Women: 27

High Blood Pressure in Black Men and White Men

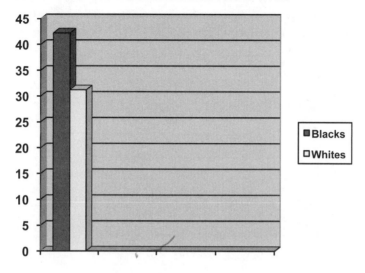

High Blood Pressure per 100,000 of population   (Source: CDC 2007)
Black Men: 42   White Men: 30

Heart Disease in Black Men and White Men

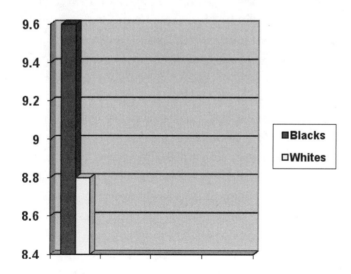

Heart Disease per 100,000 of population   (Source: CDC 2007)
Black Men: 9.6   White Men: 8.8

Heart Disease in Black Women and White Women

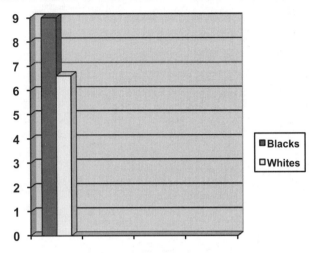

Heart Disease per 100,000 of population   (Source: CDC 2007)
Black Women: 9   White Women: 6.5

quate daily consumption of these foods can effectively address your body's calcium needs. Unfortunately, surveys show that Americans are consuming less than a third of the calcium that they need. One cup of leafy greens will supply about 300 mg of calcium, one-fourth the day's calcium need for an adult.

If you cannot satisfy your daily requirement for calcium with the foods you eat, you should take calcium supplements. In order to improve the absorption of calcium, researchers recommend that a single dose should not exceed 500 mg. Consuming more than 2000 mg of calcium per day is not recommended. Your body's need for calcium depends on your age and other physiological requirements. The table above illustrates your daily calcium requirement. Pregnant and breastfeeding women should make sure that they consume enough calcium because they need to meet the calcium needs of their young children while ensuring that their own bodies remain optimized. It is recommended that pregnant and breastfeeding mothers consume 1,000 to 1,300 mg of calcium each day. Most importantly, remember that if you take calcium supplements your intake of magnesium, vitamin D, and vitamin K2 should be optimized.

The Importance of Vitamin K2

Recent studies have found that one form of vitamin K, vitamin K2, works with vitamin D and calcium to help prevent heart disease. Whereas vitamin D helps your body to absorb calcium, studies have found that it is vitamin K2 which helps to prevent accumulation of calcium deposits in heart valves and coronary arteries by helping to direct calcium to your bones. Calcification of arteries or build-up of calcium in the arteries leads to heart disease. Without enough vitamin K2, the calcium which your body absorbs with the help of vitamin D may simply accumulate and lead to calcification of the arteries. If you are taking calcium supplements it is vital that you optimize your intake of vitamin K2. Unlike vitamin D, vitamin K2 is more readily available from food sources. Fermented soy in the form of natto, a popular food in eastern Japan, supplies the highest concentration of vitamin K2 of any food that has been measured. If you are going to consume natto you should make sure that the soy from which it is made is not genetically modified. Cheese from grass-fed animals also supplies substantial amounts of vitamin K2. If you find it difficult to obtain vitamin K2 from the food you eat, you should consider taking it in supplement form. Experts recommend that you discuss taking vitamin K2 supplements with your doctor if you are taking anticoagulant medications as K2 supplements might interfere with the role of coagulants.

Type 2 Diabetes

The number of Americans with diabetes continues to escalate at an alarming rate with the current number, approximately 24 million, estimated to be doubled in the next 25 years. Thousands of people are diagnosed with diabetes each day and blacks are disproportionately represented among diabetes sufferers. It appears that diabetes is common among blacks living in countries with high latitude and cold climates. Middle-aged blacks living in high latitude regions like Great Britain, Northern United States, and Canada suffer from type 2 diabetes at significantly higher rates than whites. Diabetes affects middle aged black women at more than twice the rate for white women. Middle aged black men also suffer disproportionately from type 2 diabetes. The National Center for Health Statistics reports that white men, 60 years and above, are more obese than black men in this age group. Obesity is a major cause of diabetes. However, black men, even with lower body weight have higher rates of diabetes. Once again it should come as no surprise because melanin in the skin works as a barrier to vitamin D production in black men.

With type 2 diabetes, your body is not able to make effective use of the insulin it produces. A person with diabetes is at risk of getting high blood pressure, vision problems, kidney disease, blood clots, amputations, and is three times more likely to die from a sudden heart attack than someone who does not have the disease. One study in a 2008 issue of the journal *Ethnicity and Disease* reports that low levels of vitamin D are found in persons with diabetes and that vitamin D deficiency could be a trigger for diabetes.

Many studies have found that people with diabetes were probably deficient in vitamin D long before physical symptoms manifested. One such study in the *Indian Journal of Medical Sciences,* involving 160 normal healthy people, found that vitamin D deficiency may cause genetic changes that create a disposition to getting diseases such as diabetes. This should serve as a warning for parents to have their children's vitamin D levels optimized and for pregnant mothers to make sure that their vitamin D levels are within normal range, between 50-80ng/ml.

Vitamin D helps the pancreas to carry out the key role of insulin secretion and use which are important factors in diabetes prevention and control. If you are diabetic, and have been taking medication without seeing any significant improvement in your condition, it may be that your body needs more vitamin D to help your cells make effective use of the insulin that is being produced in your body. An added benefit of vitamin D for diabetics is that it is an effective anti-inflammatory agent. Vitamin D is of paramount importance in the treatment of diabetes because infection levels can be quite high in the diabetic body.

Your metabolism changes as you get older but it is possible to maintain good health as you age. When you were younger, you might have been able to eat almost any kind of food without worrying how your blood sugar level would be affected. However,

Diabetes in Black Women and White Women (ages 65-74)

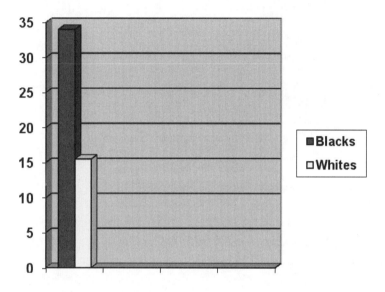

Diabetes per 100,000 of population   (Source: CDC 2007)
Black Women: 34   White Women: 15

with middle age you may notice that your blood sugar keeps moving to levels above what is considered to be normal, consequently predisposing you to a pre-diabetic state. If you are middle-aged your body cells may repair themselves more slowly and this could lead to changes in your body organs. These changes are part of the natural aging process. Healthy aging can, and should be the norm for everyone. Nutrients such as vitamin D help to prevent and control many diseases such as type 2 diabetes that are associated with aging. Type 2 diabetes can be prevented or reversed with adequate sunlight exposure, vitamin D supplementation, exercise, and a nutritious diet.

Diabetes in Black Men and White Men (ages 65-74)

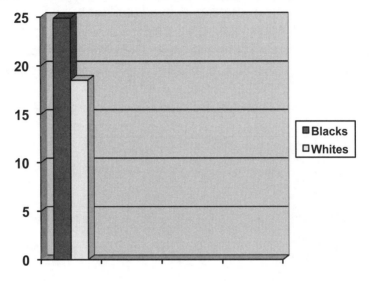

Diabetes per 100,000 of population   (Source: CDC 2007)
Black Men: 24.2   White Men: 18.7

It Is Not Only People of African Origin Who Are in Danger

Diabetes is prevalent in dark pigmented individuals and it does not matter whether you inherited your highly melanized skin from forebears who lived in Ghana, India or another region of the world. The New York City Community Health Report on diseases shows that the highest rates of diabetes are in black communities. Bangladeshi people are generally dark pigmented and this may explain why, like African Americans, they are found to be deficient in vitamin D and have higher rates of diabetes. A March 2007 issue of the journal *Diabetes, Obesity and Metabolism* reports that a London based population of Bangladeshi people had insufficient vitamin D levels in their blood and showed higher prevalence of type 2 diabetes than the white population in Britain.

Adult Obesity

The obesity epidemic is rampant in the United States, but highest among blacks. In the Fall of 2009, *Forbes Magazine* reported that one quarter of Americans suffer from obesity that will result in health care costs of $344 billion annually by 2018. The United States Centers for Disease Control and Prevention reports that significantly more blacks than whites suffer from being overweight. Sixty one percent of black women over the age of 60 are obese, and the number of overweight persons keeps increasing. It is not only elderly black women who are getting fat. More than 34 percent of American adults over the age of 20 years are obese. The Agency for Health Care Research and Quality predicts that if the current trend continues, by 2030 one half of all U.S. adults will suffer from obesity. Statistics suggest that ninety-seven percent of black women and almost the same number of Hispanics will become obese.

The obesity epidemic is cause for great concern for a number of reasons, not the least of which is the fact that overweight persons are at great risk for developing heart disease, diabetes, and many cancers. One study conducted by medical professionals at the Mercer University School of Medicine found that overweight black women have higher rates of diabetes. If this trend is not reversed the effect on the population, especially blacks, will continue to be catastrophic. Your degree of obesity depends on your body mass index (BMI) and this is calculated by dividing your weight in kilograms by your height in meters squared. If you are over 20 years of age and you have a BMI that is more than 30, you need to reduce your body fat composition.

Vitamin D Helps to Reduce Body Fat

Vitamin D works with calcium to help break down fat cells and slow the development of new fat cells. When you have insufficient vitamin D your body grows fat cells at a faster rate. Unlike vitamin D, you can often meet your calcium needs by consuming common foods. See chapters 12 and 13 for more on this. Dark-skinned people who carry too much weight face double jeopardy. Melanin constantly screens ultraviolet rays from their bodies thereby reducing vitamin D production while body fat absorbs and holds on to vitamin D making it even less available for vital immune functions. Further, as body fat increases vitamin D levels decrease, making less vitamin D available to carry out important disease prevention and lifesaving functions. Vitamin D is fat soluble so it gets absorbed into excess fat tissues. These fat tissues hold on to vitamin D and keep it sequestered so it is prevented from reaching important body targets to carry out health enhancing functions.

Obesity in Black Women and White Women (ages 40 – 59)

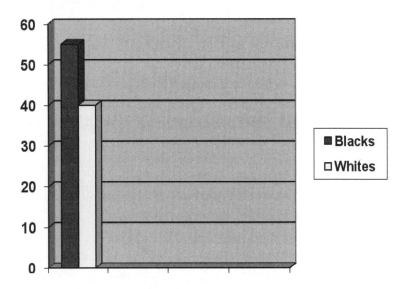

Obesity per 100,000 of population   (Source: CDC 2007)
Black Women: 55   White Women: 40

Recently, researchers established a link between vitamin D deficiency, parathyroid hormone, and obesity. Two studies conducted in 2010 found that persons deficient in vitamin D have excess parathyroid hormone levels which contribute to obesity. One of the studies, reported on in the Journal of *Clinical Endo-*

crinology, involved overweight African American adults. The study found that low vitamin D levels lead to elevated parathyroid hormone levels which, in turn, contribute to increased body fat. This finding sheds light on why many diets fail; they often do not address the underlying health conditions that may be causing obesity. There is great likelihood that if you are overweight you may have some hormonal imbalance. Dieting will not resolve

Obesity in Black Women and White Women (ages 60 and over)

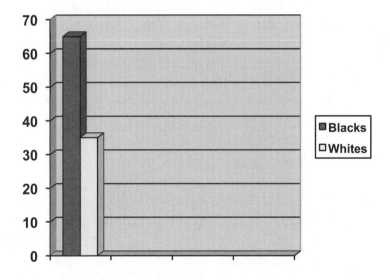

Obesity per 100,000 of population   (Source: CDC 2007)
Black Women: 61   White Women 32

these problems. However, adequate intake of vitamin D may initiate some helpful biochemical processes to help remedy these problems. Keep in mind that if you are overweight you will need to take higher daily doses of vitamin D than someone who is not overweight.

In addition to ensuring that your vitamin D levels are adequate you should make sure your diet comprises mainly nutrient-dense foods in their unaltered state, that is, not processed. It goes without saying that you should limit your sugar intake. This includes foods containing processed or refined sugars.

Childhood Obesity

Childhood obesity has been increasing at a significant rate and threatens the healthy future of one out of every three children in America. The degree of obesity in American children is quite alarming when we consider the consequences of childhood obesity. One study published in a 2004 issue of *The Journal of Clinical Endocrinology* reports that almost 70 percent of children 10 years and older who are obese will grow up to be obese adults. Obesity puts children and adults at increased risk for high cholesterol, high blood pressure, heart disease, stroke, type 2 diabetes, bone and joint problems, and several types of cancers.

Obesity related health problems in children have been increasing. During the 20 year period leading up to 2004, pediatric obesity-related hospital costs increased 3-fold, reaching $127 million per year, and this continues to increase. A 2011 report from the American Stroke Association informs us that stroke incidents are increasing among young people between the ages of 15 and 34. Many experts believe that the increase in diseases among young people is due in large part to the obesity epidemic we now face. The social and psychological problems stemming from obesity among children and our youths must also be kept in mind because children who are obese are typically stigmatized and ridiculed, which often results in poor self-image and self-esteem.

One major campaign has been aimed at reducing childhood obesity. The "Let's Move" campaign was launched by First Lady Michelle Obama to educate Americans about the causes and dangers of childhood obesity and to provide support and resources to attack childhood obesity and raise healthier Americans. You may visit the website www.letsmove.gov to get information about First Lady Michelle Obama's "Let's Move" campaign, which includes information on how you can help children eat healthy foods and engage in daily physical activities. Information about President Obama's *Healthy Hunger-Free Kids Act 2010* is also posted on the "Let's Move" website. The website www.healthieryounutrition.com and chapter 13 of this book include recipes for healthy snacks for children.

Chapter 6

Vitamin D Prevents Cancer Development and Growth

The role of vitamin D in reducing the risk of cancer has been well documented. Vitamin D from solar radiation or in supplement form has been found to have a broad spectrum preventive effect on many cancers. This nutrient, unlike cancer treatments which cost hundreds of thousands of dollars, is freely available from the sun or at very low cost from supplements. Unfortunately, many people, including blacks who have the most aggressive forms of cancer, and the highest mortality rates from cancer, are not aware of the numerous studies that have confirmed that vitamin D is effective in preventing cancer. Further, vitamin D supplementation does not carry the dangerous side effects that cancer drugs are known to cause.

Current cancer research informs us that vitamin D may help prevent 2 million cancer deaths each year. Cancers of the pancreas, lung and prostate gland are a few of the types of cancers that may be prevented with vitamin D. When one considers the deadly nature of cancer cells it is nothing short of a medical feat to use vitamin D to stimulate self-destruction of cancerous cells, reduce their spread and retard the growth of new blood vessels that carry nourishment to cancer cells. Pancreatic cancer is not only difficult to diagnose but has a low survival rate. When compared to the death rate from other cancers lung cancer carries the highest mortality rate among blacks. African American men have the highest mortality rates from both lung and prostate cancers.

Vitamin D Works with Calcium to Prevent Cancer

Like other nutrients, vitamin D works with cofactors to carry out its important metabolic functions. In 2007, a study published in the *American Journal of Clinical Nutrition* confirmed what epidemiological cancer studies have been showing for decades. The researchers in this study set up a double blind, randomized placebo-controlled investigation and the study confirmed that vitamin D works with calcium to substantially reduce cancer risks. This four-year population based study involving women above the age of 55 years found that improved nutritional status of vitamin D and calcium helps to prevent all forms of cancer.

Season when Cancer Is Diagnosed Influences Outcomes

Studies have found that the season in which diagnosis of cancer is done influences a patient's prognosis. Cancer patients tend to live longer if the cancer is diagnosed in summer as opposed to winter. During the winter months the hours of sunlight are very short and scientists report that even if you sit in the sun all day, from November to March in northern regions above 35 degrees latitude, you get almost no vitamin D from the sun. Regions of the United States that fall above 35 degrees latitude include places positioned north of Atlanta, Georgia.

Far too many incidents of dark-skinned people succumbing to chronic diseases especially during winter months occur. In one such incident a 49-year-old dark-skinned medical doctor who was diagnosed with cancer during the winter in New York City died within one week of being admitted to the hospital. He did not die because of poor access to health care, inadequate access to fresh foods or because his education was below standard. It is quite likely that he succumbed to cancer because his dark skin reduced his body's vitamin D production and he did not compensate by taking supplements. The deceased medical doctor maintained a healthy diet, normal weight and a healthy appearance but he did not take vitamin D supplements. In *The Vitamin D Revolution,* Dr. Soram Khalsa explains that patients who fit this profile yet still develop cancer, usually have low vitamin D levels.

An examination of geographical distribution of cancer cases reveals the crucial role which vitamin D plays in preventing cancer. African American women who live in the sunshine states have lower breast cancer rates than those living in sunlight poor states. Black men living in sunny climates also have lower rates of prostate cancer than those who live in sunlight poor areas. However, keep in mind that even if you live in a sunlight rich area you still need to get in the sun and stay under the rays of sunlight for a few hours every day in order to help prevent cancer and other diseases. If being in the sun for a few hours daily isn't feasible for you, it is imperative that you take vitamin D supplements.

Breast Cancer

Vitamin D has been proven to be extremely effective against breast cancer. In one study carried out at the State University of New York, cancer cells of the breast withered and died within a few days of being injected with a potent form of vitamin D.

Breast cancer is more aggressive in dark-skinned women and scientists believe that vitamin D deficiency in black women is a major cause for the aggressive course that breast cancer takes in black women. A study published in a 2009 issue of the *Journal of Clinical Oncology* found that a high percentage of premenopausal women from the Northeastern United States diagnosed with breast cancer were deficient in vitamin D. The recommended measurement of vitamin D for optimal health, ranges between 50ng/ml and 100ng/ml, but participants in this study had vitamin D levels below 20ng/ml. The black women in the study had the greatest vitamin D deficiency. After one year of getting the then recommended daily allowance of 400 IU of vitamin D, and 1,000 mg of calcium, the participants in the study were tested again. Less than 15 percent of the white and Hispanic women had vitamin D levels considered to be normal, but none of the black women had vitamin D levels that were considered healthy.

Black women also have a lower survival rate for breast cancer. Data from the American Cancer Society reveals that 90 percent of white women with breast cancer live to the long term survival mark but only 76 percent of black women live to this mark. Women who live for 20 to 30 years after cancer diagnosis are said to be long term survivors. One study in the April 2009 issue of *Annals of Epidemiology*, reports that women with blood vitamin D levels higher than 29 ng/ml had about 50 percent less metastases than women with lower levels. According to this report, women with higher levels of vitamin D were also more likely to be long term cancer survivors. Another study in the September 2008 issue of the *Journal of the National Medical Association* found that black women have a 50 percent greater risk of dying from breast cancer, after adjusting for locality, treatment, and hormone status.

Triple-Negative Breast Cancer

The incidence rate of triple-negative breast cancer, an extremely aggressive form of breast cancer, is very high among black women. Researchers have found that black women from diverse ethnicities have triple negative breast cancer at a rate of three times the rate for non-black women. Triple negative is so named because it lacks receptors for three hormones that are usually targeted by cancer drugs. This type of cancer affects young as well as older black women, but is most often found in younger black women. It affects women regardless of their body mass, and it is common in obese as well as non-obese black women. Triple negative carries a poor prognosis because it has a greater number of metastases, and typically kills its victim in an average time of three years. Researchers in one study found that triple negative breast cancer patients had significantly lower vitamin D levels than the normal study population.

Breast Cancer Death Rates in Blacks and Whites

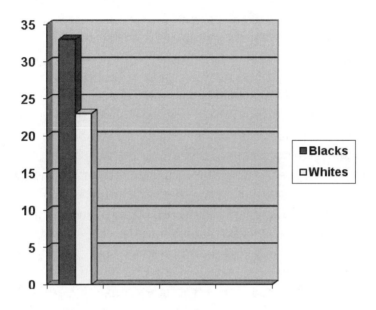

Breast Cancer Death Rate per 100,000 of population   (Source: CDC 2007)
Blacks: 33   Whites: 23

Lung Cancer

Lung cancer is the leading cause of cancer related deaths in America. African American men, who bear the greatest burden of this disease, are 37 percent more likely than white men to get lung cancer and 22 percent more likely to die from it. The incidence of lung cancer among black women is roughly similar to that for white women.

Lung cancer occurs as a result of rapid, uncontrolled growth of abnormal cells in the lungs. There are two main types of lung cancer: non small cell lung cancer (NSCLC) and small cell lung cancer (SCLC). Non small cell lung cancer is the more common type, accounting for approximately 85 percent of all lung cancer cases. Non small cell lung cancer usually develops slowly and spreads to different parts of the body more slowly than small cell lung cancer. It usually goes undetected for long periods of time and quite often is not diagnosed until it is very advanced. Small cell lung cancer on the other hand, grows and spreads more rapidly to other areas of the body.

Although lung cancer is usually associated with smoking, black men who smoke at almost the same levels as white men are far more likely to get and die from lung cancer than whites. One major study, which examined the differences in risk for lung cancer among different ethnic groups, found that the higher susceptibility of blacks to lung cancer could not be explained by differences in socioeconomic status. In this study, African Americans, despite having some college education, were still more likely to get lung cancer. These disparities in lung cancer rates do not only apply to smokers. A 2008 study with 1.8 million self-reported never-smokers found that African Americans ages 40-84 were more likely to get and die from lung cancer than the participants who were of European descent.

No large-scale study investigating the huge disparities in risk of lung cancer among various ethnic groups has examined the role of vitamin D deficiency in the incidence and mortality rates of lung cancer. However, a number of studies have found that vitamin D can mitigate the growth of lung cancer cells. A study reported on in a 2007 issue of the *Journal of Clinical Oncology* found that the vitamin D status of a lung cancer patient, before and at the time of diagnosis, is an important factor in lung cancer survival. Data collected from 447 patients with early stage lung cancer, linked overall survival of patients with high levels of vitamin D circulating in the body.

Other studies examining the role of vitamin D in the survival rates of early stage non small cell lung cancer patients have found that those with higher vitamin D levels had higher survival times than other patients with lower vitamin D intake. The studies also found that higher vitamin D levels may be associated with less aggressive development of lung cancer that is diagnosed in its early stages. Further, researchers have also observed significant associations between vitamin D levels and the season during which surgery is performed. Early stage non small cell lung cancer patients with higher vitamin D levels who had surgery during the summer months had significantly improved survival rates than patients who had surgery during the winter months with lower vitamin D levels. Based on these findings, researchers recommend that early stage lung cancer patients, and especially those who tend to be deficient in vitamin D, supplement with vitamin D particularly in the winter months.

Lung Cancer in Black Men and White Men

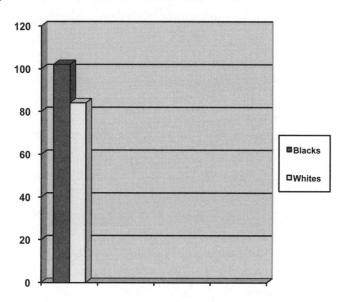

Lung Cancer per 100,000 of the population (Source: CDC 2007)
Black Men: 102   White Men: 84

Colorectal Cancer

Colorectal cancer, cancer of the colon or rectum, is the second leading cause of cancer related deaths. African Americans have the highest incidence and mortality rates from colorectal cancer in the United States with black men suffering the most fatalities from it. What exactly is colorectal cancer or colon cancer as it is commonly referred to and how is it formed?

Your colon is part of your large intestine. It is a long tube approximately 5 feet long which goes up the right side of your abdomen (the ascending colon), across your abdomen (the transverse colon), and down the left side of your abdomen (the descending colon). It merges with the rectum at its lower portion.

Your colon facilitates an extremely important function in the digestive process by absorbing water from undigested food and helping to form stool for elimination. As a site of fermentation, the colon has multiple types of bacteria in large numbers which aid the breakdown of food and help to prevent the overgrowth of harmful bacteria. A properly functioning colon must be very efficient at moving waste material. Problems typically arise when the movement of waste through the large intestine is hindered.

Efficient movement of food through your intestines in conjunction with stomach and bile acids and digestive enzymes help to reduce the likelihood that harmful bacteria will proliferate in your colon. However, the average time that food sits in your colon and rectum before it is expelled is two days. Consequently, if harmful bacteria present in your food at time of ingestion are not destroyed before they enter your small intestine, chances are they will begin to grow and proliferate in your colon as your food sits waiting to be expelled. Needless to say, the longer waste products from digestion sit in your colon before being expelled as fecal waste, and the more harmful bacteria you have in your colon and rectum, the greater the chances of toxic build up from disease promoting bacteria and possibly cancer. Harmful bacteria in the colon contribute to ongoing inflammation and speed up the colonic cell life cycle thus predisposing you to cancer.

Studies have shown that vitamin D stimulates the production of substances which help to kill harmful organisms and prevent inflammation in the intestines. One study led by Dr. Vin Tangpricha, professor at Emory University School of Medicine, found that colon cancer develops faster in people who are deficient in vitamin D. A study reported on in a 2010 issue of the

British Medical Journal found that blood measurements of vitamin D between 50 to 75 nmol/L, decreases ones chance of getting colorectal cancer, and levels of vitamin D that are higher than 75 nmol/L, were associated with even lower colorectal cancer risk. This study also found that higher consumption of calcium in the diet plays a significant role in preventing colon cancer.

Many studies have shown that diet influences your risk of developing colon cancer perhaps more so than any other type of cancer. Diets high in refined carbohydrates, processed meats, and low in fiber rich vegetables and fruits increase your chances of developing cancer in general but especially colon cancer. Eating fiber rich vegetables is especially important for maintaining a healthy digestive tract as these act much like a scrubbing brush aiding the digestive process by "cleaning" the intestinal walls and moving food efficiently through the intestines, thus facilitating rapid transit.

In addition to maintaining adequate vitamin D levels and a healthy diet, it is also important to get regular colonoscopy screenings as a preventative measure against colon cancer.

Colorectal Cancer in Black Men and White Men

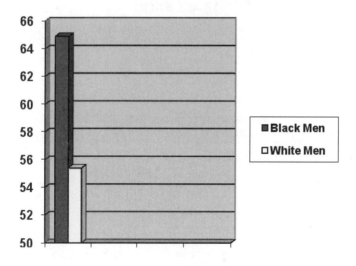

Rate per 100,000 of population (Source: CDC 2007)
Black Men: 65   White Men: 55

Colorectal Cancer in Black Women and White Women

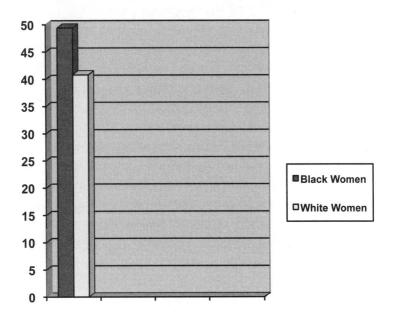

Rate per 100,000 of population   (Source: CDC 2007)
Black Women: 50   White Women 41

Prostate Cancer

Prostate cancer is the second leading cause of death from cancer among men. Men with African ancestry are most susceptible to getting prostate cancer and dying from it. African Americans have an incidence rate of prostate cancer that is up to three times more than Caucasian Americans. Unlike other cancers with geographical patterns that provide strong support for the beneficial role of UVB radiation, the incidence rate of prostate cancer varies from state to state in the United States with the most concentrated regions in the Northwestern states. For these reasons, researchers believe that both genetics and diet are factors in the prevalence of prostate cancer among men with African ancestry. One gene in particular, known as ApoE4, has been implicated in the incidence of prostate cancer and some studies have identified its prevalence among men with African ancestry in many countries around the world. Diet has also been implicated in prostate cancer incidence rates. Some studies have found that adoption of Westernized diets has been associated with increased risk for prostate cancer. In general, lowfat/non-fat milk and animal products have been associated with increased risk for prostate cancer while vegetables have been associated with reduced risk. High cholesterol and inflammation also increase one's risk of getting prostate cancer.

Some studies have found that adequate vitamin D levels can reduce your risk of developing prostate cancer. Vitamin D helps to prevent unrestrained cell division and multiplication that may lead to cancer of the prostate. In one study from the Harvard School of Public Health, vitamin D levels of approximately 3,000 men, some of whom had prostate cancer, were examined. Researchers found that those with higher levels of vitamin D in

Prostate Cancer in Black Men and White Men

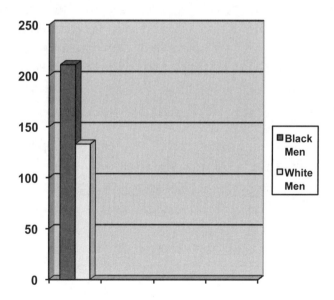

Prostate Cancer per 100,000 of population   (Source: CDC 2007)
Black Men: 210   White Men: 133

their blood were less likely to get prostate cancer. Similarly, a study reported on in the April 2009 issue of *Annals of Epidemiology* found that men who were 57 years of age and older displayed a very low risk of getting prostate cancer when their blood vitamin D levels were above 28 ng/ml. The study also found that men whose vitamin D levels were below 28 ng/ml had twice the incidence of aggressive prostate cancer. Another study reported on in the journal of *Alternative Therapies* found that men with prostate cancer who were given vitamin D daily over a twenty-one month period were able to reduce their PSA level by 50 percent.

Several studies have shown that vitamin D can reduce the severity of prostate cancer and increase survival for prostate cancer patients. Vitamin D helps to slow the growth of prostate cancer cells and promote the growth of healthy prostate cells. Vitamin D also helps with proper utilization of calcium, excesses of which have been implicated in prostate cancer in some studies. When there is not enough vitamin D to help the body to make effective use of calcium, blood levels of calcium can accumulate and contribute to the development of prostate cancer. Researchers in a U.S. government health survey tracked 2,814 men and found that high levels of serum calcium increased their risk of developing prostate cancer.

If you are a middle-aged dark skinned man you can minimize your risk of developing prostate cancer by eating a healthy diet with lots of vegetables, ensuring that your vitamin D levels are adequate, and getting screened for prostate cancer.

Chapter 7

Mood Disorders

Vitamin D Deficiency Is Associated with Mental Illness

Recent studies have linked low vitamin D levels to depression and mood problems. Vitamin D and its nutrition co-factors can help to stabilize mood. You may be familiar with the bothersome behaviors of children who will sit still and concentrate for short periods of time only. Studies show that vitamin D is involved in normal brain development and others indicate that some black youngsters develop depression, attention deficit hyperactive disorder, and other mood problems partly due to low vitamin D levels.

Schizophrenia Risk among Blacks Linked to Vitamin D Deficiency

Recent studies involving populations in the United States, Norway, and the Netherlands have established a link between vitamin D deficiency and depression. Vitamin D deficiency is also associated with more serious cases of mental illness such as bipolar disorder and schizophrenia. Critical deficiency in vitamin D places blacks at greater risk of developing these conditions. One study in a 2009 issue of *Nutrition Reviews* found that schizophrenia was observed to be more common in dark-skinned migrants to northwestern Europe. Other studies show that dark-skinned people who migrate from African and Caribbean countries to colder Northern countries, located at higher latitudes, often succumb to schizophrenia and other mental illnesses. A recent study found that black immigrants to the United States are at very high risk for developing schizophrenia. Studies carried out in Finland showed that there was a reduced risk of schizophrenia in those who were given vitamin D supplementation during the first year of life.

One study published in *The Journal of Psychiatry and Neuroscience* questions whether the time has come for clinical trials to be done on vitamin D as an antidepressant. Testing the vitamin D levels of psychiatric patients and supplementing them with vitamin D would be a wise and inexpensive move for hospitals to make. Treatment teams at psychiatric hospitals may need to give patients, especially dark-skinned persons, daily dosages of more than 5,000 International Units of vitamin D for a number of reasons. First, scientific studies have shown that dark-skinned people are critically low in vitamin D and that this deficiency often contributes to schizophrenia. Equally important, hospitalized patients are locked away from sunlight so hospitalization further depletes the vitamin D that patients may have had before they were hospitalized. Additionally, psychiatric drugs leech vitamin D from the bodies of patients, causing these sick people to become even more vitamin D deficient. A therapeutic daily dosage of vitamin D for black psychiatric patients may prevent them from becoming sicker. The health preserving function of vitamin D may help to reduce the toxic effects and dangerous side effects of psychiatric drug cocktails.

The human body is a marvelous machine that can often fix itself once it gets the proper fuel to run on, so people with depression or mood problems need not despair. They should seek help and try to have the problem addressed without the use of pharmaceutical drugs. If it is necessary to use prescription drugs, patients should not stop taking these drugs abruptly. Instead, people who use depression medication should work with medical personnel who understand that natural substances play very important roles in the biochemical functioning of the body. With the help of medical personnel, prescription medication may be reduced to a minimum amount and gradually eliminated.

Do You Have Chronic Body Pain?

Chronic pain is so prevalent in the United States that pain management is practiced as a medical specialty. Almost 20 percent of adults in the United States suffer from chronic pain of the muscles and bones and the most common of these is felt in the back. The United States Centers for Disease Control and Prevention (CDC) reports that 16 million Americans are limited in their physical activities due to arthritis. However, a greater number of blacks than whites have limited physical activity and severe joint pain as a result of arthritis. Frequent complaints of body pain may be caused from osteoarthritis, bone disease and other conditions, but research and modern medicine have pointed to a psychological cause of many cases of chronic pain in multiple locations of the body.

Musculoskeletal pain (pain in the muscles and bones) is often caused by a condition known as fibromyalgia. This is also called nerve pain. Fibromyalgia has been linked to depression and anxiety that result from emotional trauma. Sleep disturbance may worsen this condition. Fibromyalgia is also linked to vitamin D deficiency and vitamin D supplementation can be used to treat this condition. Vitamin D works with nutrients such as magnesium and calcium to prevent and alleviate pain in the muscles and bones. Magnesium supplementation can raise your pain threshold by making your body less sensitive to pain, while this mineral works with vitamin D and calcium to repair musculoskeletal problems that cause the pain.

Fibromyalgia is often confused with osteomalacia. Osteo-malacia is also known as adult rickets because, like rickets in children, it is caused from vitamin D deficiency and inadequate mineralization of the bones. Faulty or inadequate bone mineral deposits lead to bending of the bones and bone pain. The bending or bowing of weak bones can also place undue stress on the muscles of the body.

Vitamin D Supplementation Relieves Chronic Pain

Linda, a 70-year-old dark-skinned female listened to one of my nutrition presentations on the role of vitamin D in the body. At the end of the presentation she indicated that she was familiar with vitamin D and shared her experience on vitamin D. She suffered from aches and pain throughout her body and visited many doctors for many years in an attempt to get relief, but she was not able to reduce her suffering despite taking numerous medications that were prescribed by the doctors she visited. Fortunately, someone advised Linda to visit a physician who integrates natural treatments in her medical protocol. Linda explained that the pain in her bones and muscles were so intense that she was willing to try any treatment that was different from the ones that she had been receiving. The vitamin D treatment that her integrative physician prescribed for her brought her so much relief that she keeps this supplement in her purse to make sure it is always on hand wherever she goes. She explained that her doctor advised her to take 50,000 IU of vitamin D per week for eight weeks, after which time she would have her vitamin D level tested and her dosage of vitamin D reduced to a lower daily maintenance amount.

Chapter 8

Special Vitamin D Needs of Elderly Dark-Skinned People and Institutionalized Persons Who Are Dark-Skinned

Dark-skinned people who are elderly as well as dark-skinned people who are institutionalized have special vitamin D needs. Factors such as advanced age and being institutionalized can have significant adverse effects on one's health. Dark skin pigmentation, advanced age, and being institutionalized present significant barriers to effective vitamin D production and utilization. Each of these conditions can pose significant threats to optimum health. However, any combination of these conditions may result in even more health risks.

Unique Vitamin D Needs of Elderly Dark-Skinned People

More than 50 percent of the general U.S. population over the age of 65 has been found deficient in vitamin D. Aging causes body cells, tissues, and organs to be less efficient in vitamin D production and other functioning. A seventy-five year old person can produce only 25 percent of the vitamin D that a twenty-five year-old produces. This places elderly people at great risk for developing diseases such as diabetes, heart disease, and cancer. The combined risks of dark skin pigmentation and advanced age place elderly blacks at even greater risk for developing these diseases. Elderly dark-skinned people who are in nursing homes or other institutionalized settings may not be getting adequate sunlight exposure and may therefore have even greater vitamin D requirements.

Adequate vitamin D modifies dangerous health conditions that are associated with aging such as insulin resistance and inflammation. In healthy people, insulin, a hormone that is produced by the pancreas, carries out a number of important metabolic functions. One of these is the regulation of blood sugar levels. Insulin facilitates the passage of glucose from the blood to cells of the body to produce energy and carry out life sustaining processes. When there is a fault in the insulin regulation system, the body fails to keep blood sugar levels normal and diabetes typically develops. The body struggles to get rid of excess blood sugar that under normal circumstances would be used for energy. Blood sugar or glucose therefore gets spilled into the urine. This causes frequent urination, excessive thirst and extra work for the kidneys. These are some of the symptoms of diabetes, and when unchecked, diabetes can cause damage to the kidneys, heart, eyes and nerves. By effecting proper insulin signaling, vitamin D plays an important role in preventing and arresting the dangerous health conditions that usually stem from faulty insulin regulation.

Vitamin D and Physical Functioning in Elderly Dark-Skinned People

Very few studies exist on the unique vitamin D needs of elderly people who are dark-skinned. However, researchers have found that vitamin D deficiency in older African Americans has been associated with lower bone mineral density of the hip. *The Journal of the American Medical Association* reports that African Americans are more deficient in vitamin D and tend to have more hip fractures than whites. The mortality rate from osteoporotic fractures is also greater in blacks than whites. Elderly men and women with low vitamin D in their blood score lower on physical performance tests than those who have adequate vitamin D in their blood. Insulin is a powerful hormone that works with vitamin D to enhance muscle and bone strength.

I talked with an elderly dark-skinned woman who was misdiagnosed because her vitamin D deficiency was confused with other conditions. She had deep gnawing pain in her bones and muscles all over her body and several doctors placed her on medication for many different complaints. Fortunately for her, a physician later diagnosed her vitamin D deficiency and prescribed 50,000 IU of vitamin D per week for 8 weeks. She now takes a lower daily maintenance dose of vitamin D and has no pain or weakness in her muscles and bones.

Vitamin D also works with calcium to produce strong bones and teeth. We should not forget that elderly people can also have strong, efficient, and attractive teeth even as they age. *Public Health Nutrition* reports that calcium and vitamin D help to reduce tooth loss in the elderly. Of course, elderly people with dark skin are in the greatest danger because of their highly melanized skin. It is therefore very important that caregivers ensure that vitamin D levels of elderly blacks are kept optimized.

Vitamin D and Mental Function in Elderly Dark-Skinned People

Dementia, reduced mental functioning, and Alzheimer's disease are conditions which many of us have come to associate with aging. The good news is that research has shown that natural UVB rays of the sun, vitamin D supplementation, and bright light therapy can reorder circadian rhythm functioning, correct sleep patterns, and improve mental functioning. Vitamin D has far-reaching positive effects on the brain and may prevent decline in mental functioning in the elderly. A study reported on in a July 2010 issue of *The Archive of Internal Medicine* found that low levels of vitamin D were associated with substantial cognitive decline in elderly persons. A total of 858 persons 65 years and older were examined over a six year period. Participants in the study were interviewed, given cognitive assessments, and had medical examinations done. Those with adequate levels of vitamin D performed better on the assessments and were more mentally astute than participants with low vitamin D levels.

The importance of optimum vitamin D levels for effective mental functioning has also been confirmed by other studies. A University of Manchester study found that men over the age of 60 with adequate blood levels of vitamin D have better visual memory and greater information processing speed. *The Journal of the National Medical Association* reported that among older African Americans, vitamin D deficiency is associated with impaired cognitive performance. Some researchers have also found that vitamin D helps to relieve depression and reduce the risk of dementia in the elderly, and have suggested that vitamin D supplementation be used as a safe low-cost preventative treatment for brain disorders in the elderly. One study reported on in the *Journal of Alzheimer's Disease* found that there is evidence that vitamin D reduces the risk of many diseases that often lead to dementia. There is hope that optimized vitamin D levels may help to prevent the decline in cognitive functions that have come to be associated with aging.

Special Vitamin D Needs of Hospitalized Blacks

People who are institutionalized have greater vitamin D requirements because of limited sunlight exposure. In addition to having limited sunlight exposure, people who are hospitalized have additional vitamin D requirements because of the many infections which are notorious for being transmitted in hospital settings. Hospital patients are also in great danger of dying from these hospital-acquired infections. According to the CDC, approximately 2 million Americans contracted infections during their stay in hospitals in 2007 and 100,000 people died from these infections. A recent study reported on in *Academy Emergency Medicine* found that vitamin D deficiency is associated with increased infection rates among hospital patients. Dark-skinned people who are predisposed to chronic vitamin D deficiency outside of hospitalization face even more serious health threats if they are not supplemented with vitamin D while they are hospitalized.

Vitamin D plays an important role in inflammation prevention from surgical or other wounds and helps the immune system to fight off hospital-acquired germs. Methicillin-resistant Staphylococcus aureus (MRSA) is a highly transmittable bacterial germ which has been quietly killing people for decades and is often found in hospitals. MRSA infections kill more people than HIV/AIDS. *The Journal of the American Medical Association* reports that there were approximately 100,000 MRSA infections in the United States in 2005 and these infections continue to pose great danger. Vitamin D acts as a natural antibiotic and protects the body against infectious diseases such as those that may be associated with MRSA.

The immune system of hospitalized patients may be strengthened with vitamin D in order to guard against another dangerous form of bacteria that has emerged in hospitals, *Clostridium difficile (C. difficile)*. *C. difficile* spores are prolific and resistant. These spores generally spread to new victims from the hands of health care workers and they can live for months or years on contaminated surfaces while resisting many disinfectants. The prolific nature of *C. difficile* is seen in the great number of this organism excreted in diarrhea from feces. Each gram of fecal excrement carries 10,000 to 10 million *C. difficile.* Persons who are elderly, immune-compromised, and persons who take broad scope antibiotic medications are in greater danger of getting sick or dying from *C. difficile infection.* A recent study done on community hospitals in Georgia, North Carolina, South Carolina, and Virginia, found that infection rates from *Clostridium difficile* was 25 percent higher than infections from MRSA. Hospitalization may be necessary for different reasons, and hospitalization may save your life, but your hospital stay may also pose additional problems to your health and even shorten your life. It is highly recommended that medical personnel ensure that blood vitamin D levels of all patients, especially blacks, are optimized.

Dark-Skinned Patients in Psychiatric Hospitals Need High Dosage Vitamin D

Patients who are hospitalized in psychiatric facilities often suffer from vitamin D deficiency. Vitamin D aids the process of absorption of calcium and helps to transport calcium and phosphorus to bones and other parts of the body. Vitamin D also works with magnesium to carry out hundreds of biological activities in the body. When magnesium, calcium and vitamin D are absorbed in the body, one of the effects is especially immediate and remarkable. There is usually relief from muscle pain. Mentally ill people often complain of body pain, and muscle pain is usually among the battery of illnesses that result from psychological trauma and anxiety. Along with chronic pain, many psychiatric patients also suffer from decreased muscle strength, an illness that is attributable to vitamin D deficiency. Heavily melanized skin, lack of sunlight, and a cocktail of psychiatric drugs can place dark-skinned psychiatric patients at great risk of becoming sicker when they are hospitalized. Psychiatric drugs are known to lower the blood levels of vitamin D and other nutrients. Mentally ill people, especially those with dark skin, need to take vitamin D supplements in high dosages.

Special Vitamin D Needs of Dark-Skinned Incarcerated Persons

Like other institutionalized persons, people who are incarcerated have special vitamin D needs because of decreased sunlight exposure and little if any vitamin D supplementation. This issue has special significance for dark-skinned persons because of the disproportionate number of blacks who are incarcerated in American prisons. The United States prison population stands at 1.5 million inmates, with state and federal prisons above capacity by 16 percent and 39 percent, respectively. The black prison population represents a significant percentage of the total prison population in the U.S. In 2007, 92 percent of the U.S. prison population was male and according to national records, the incarceration rate for black males was 4, 618 per 100,000, Hispanic males were incarcerated at 1,747 per 100,000, and white males at 773 per 100,000.

Chapter 9

Special Vitamin D Needs of Dark-Skinned Pregnant and Lactating Women and Dark-Skinned Children

Vitamin D has such profound influence on development during the early years and on one's risk of developing certain cancers and autoimmune diseases later in life that it is imperative that special attention be given to the unique vitamin D requirements of dark-skinned pregnant and lactating women and young children who are darkly pigmented. Inadequate vitamin D levels during the early years predispose one to a host of chronic and degenerative diseases later in life.

Pregnant women who are deficient in vitamin D face many health risks including pre-eclampsia, anemia, spontaneous pre-term birth, gestational diabetes, greater risk of primary cesarean section, and even death during child-birth. Among other researchers, Dr. Bruce Hollis has for many years called attention to the woefully inadequate Recommended Daily Allowance (RDA) for the unique vitamin D needs of pregnant and lactating women. Young children with insufficient vitamin D are at risk of developing a host of chronic diseases including rickets, frequent colds and respiratory infections, eczema, and attention deficit hyperactivity disorder (ADHD), to name a few. This vitamin D insufficiency during the early years sets the stage for developing a number of diseases later in life, including cancers, high blood pressure, and schizophrenia. It is important to note that pregnant women who have insufficient vitamin D levels during pregnancy usually pass on their vitamin D deficiency status to their children.

By optimizing her vitamin D levels, a pregnant mother is taking an important health-enhancing and life-saving step for both herself and her child. Experts have found that pregnant mothers who supplement with 4,000 IU of vitamin D daily cut their risk of having a pre-term birth by half. Pregnant women with adequate vitamin D levels also experience fewer infections, fewer cases of gestational diabetes, less likelihood of developing anemia, have fewer primary cesarian sections, reduced incidence of high blood pressure, and fewer cases of pre-eclampsia.

Ensuring adequate vitamin D levels during pregnancy is also especially important because without sufficient vitamin D, calcium cannot be properly absorbed and utilized by the body. This is of extreme significance during pregnancy because during pregnancy a woman's need for calcium is almost double that of a man of the same age. A woman's calcium stores are called upon during pregnancy to help build the bones of her developing fetus and young child. Without enough absorption of calcium a pregnant woman's bones will deteriorate and the skeletal structure of her newborn will not be well developed. This of course, leads to conditions such as rickets.

Since vitamin D is so critical to optimal growth and development it is imperative that all dark-skinned women of childbearing age ensure that their vitamin D levels are optimized. Black mothers may need more than 4,000 IU of vitamin D because melanin in the skin serves as a barrier to adequate vitamin D production from the sun.

High Incidence of Vitamin D Deficiency in Pregnant Dark-Skinned Women

Vitamin D deficiency is widespread among pregnant women but extremely high in black pregnant women. African American women are significantly more deficient in vitamin D than white women and their risk of having pre-term birth, pre-eclampsia, and other adverse conditions associated with pregnancy are greater than those for white women.

Researchers at the University of Pittsburg, School of Public Health collected blood samples from 400 first time mothers at the beginning of their pregnancy and again at the end of pregnancy. Half the women were black and half were white. More than half the participants took multivitamins that contained vitamin D during pregnancy, and many took multivitamins before becoming pregnant. Not surprisingly, at the time of delivery only 4 percent of the black women had vitamin D levels considered sufficient for good health. Needless to say, multivitamins are an inadequate source for addressing vitamin D needs. This is especially so for black women who need far more than the recommended daily allowance of vitamin D to maintain adequate vitamin D levels and good health.

Vitamin D Deficiency Alters Gene Expression

Vitamin D deficiency before birth can alter gene expression. With vitamin D deficiency so prevalent among pregnant black women, it is plausible that this deficiency adversely affects the developing brains of many black children. One study led by a criminologist at a Florida University found that certain dopamine gene variations are linked to brain dysfunction. Brain malfunction can lead to behaviors such as attention deficit hyperactivity disorder (ADHD). Unfortunately, this study did not examine the role that vitamin D might have played in gene alteration. It is quite possible that chronic vitamin D deficiency might have led to altered genes in many of the black children placed in special education classes. However, the good news is that genes do not have to predetermine anyone's fate in life. You can take proactive steps to ensure good health. Ensuring that a developing fetus and young children have adequate vitamin D levels and proper nutrition can help correct genetic predispositions for certain diseases later in life.

Vitamin D and Gender Bender Chemicals

Researchers have found that women who are exposed to substances known as phthalates are at increased risk for giving birth to pre-term babies. It is believed that these chemicals cause intrauterine inflammation and pre-term birth. Phthalates have also been found to reduce testosterone synthesis and may result in incomplete testicular descent in boys. Pregnant women need to be very aware of these substances that may affect their unborn children.

It is difficult to avoid breathing polluted air, drinking water that has chemicals and eating pesticide laden foods. However, maintaining optimal vitamin D levels facilitates the natural detoxification process in our bodies. Vitamin D detoxifies the body by increasing glutathione levels. Glutathione is a detoxifying agent which helps to remove many dangerous chemicals such as drugs and environmental pollutants from the body. One recent study found that even mercury can be removed from the body when cells are optimally supplied with vitamin D.

Some of the dangerous substances that affect reproductive health are found in plastic containers, wrappings, household chemicals, utensils and gadgets, processed food packaging, lubricant and adhesives, detergents, nail polish, hair spray, shampoo, deodorants and fragrances and toys, vinyl flooring and wall covering. Other endocrine disrupters are the food additive monosodium glutamate (MSG), insecticides and herbicides used to spray vegetables and fruits, artificial growth hormones used to produce milk and meat, teflon coating inside pots and pans, and resins lining some food cans.

Black women and young black children are most at risk of being exposed to toxic endocrine disruptors and other environmental pollutants. Studies have found that lower income people often live in highly polluted neighborhoods. African-Americans comprise a disproportionate percentage of lower income people who live in toxic neighborhoods where environmental conditions violate the Clean Air and Clean Water Pact. One laboratory test commissioned by the *Environmental Working*

Group found more than 200 dangerous chemicals in the cord blood of African American, Asian and Hispanic newborns. Needless to say, this is cause for great concern because many of these babies who have been found to have high levels of dangerous chemicals in their blood are also born without sufficient levels of vitamin D to help counteract the adverse effects of this pollution. It cannot be emphasized enough that pregnant black mothers optimize their vitamin D levels.

Pre-eclampsia and Vitamin D

Pre-eclampsia, low birth weight, and high infant mortality rates are prevalent among blacks. Pre-eclampsia or toxemia of pregnancy usually shows up after the 20th week of pregnancy. The mother's blood pressure rises and protein is usually found in her urine. Pre-eclampsia can seriously affect the mother's kidney, liver, and brain, endangers both mother and child, causes low birth weight, premature birth, stillbirth and sometimes death of the mother. In fact, pre-eclampsia is the second leading cause of mother's death during pregnancy and it is often caused by low vitamin D in the mother's blood. One study published in *Nutrition Reviews* found that pre-eclamptic placentas might have decreased ability to convert vitamin D to its active form. Adequate vitamin D supplementation can reduce the risk of pre-eclampsia. In Finland, the risk of pre-eclampsia was cut by half in women who received vitamin D supplementation during the first year of their own childhood.

Raising Birth Weight and Lowering Infant Mortality

Statistics from the *March of Dimes* show that as many as 543,000 babies or one out of every eight babies born in the U.S. is a result of pre-mature birth each year. The United States has a pre-mature birth rate that is higher than most other developed countries. Babies who weigh less than five and a half pounds or 2500 grams are said to have very low birth weight (VLBW). Studies have found that African-American women are approximately three times more likely than white women to give birth to VLBW babies. These infants often have underdeveloped organs which can impede their health and progress in life. More than 50 percent of blacks are deficient in vitamin D during the reproductive years and this deficiency contributes significantly to VLBW babies.

Besides the disadvantages mentioned above, VLBW babies tend to have low survival rates. This amounts to a high infant mortality rate that is even higher among African-American teen-agers. At birth a baby is thoroughly examined and given a health score called an Apgar score. Low birth weight babies tend to have low Apgar scores which suggest that these babies may face significant health problems. Since vitamin D plays such an important role in the pre-natal development of babies and children's health, it is quite clear that vitamin D deficiency among dark-skinned people is partly responsible for the high incidence of low birth weight and high infant mortality rates seen among blacks.

Higher Vitamin D Levels May Reduce the Risk of HIV Transmission from Mothers to Children

The Journal of Infectious Diseases reports that HIV positive pregnant mothers with insufficient vitamin D place their unborn children at greater risk. HIV positive mothers with low vitamin D levels increase the risk of passing HIV to their babies. Eight hundred and eighty-four HIV positive Tanzanian women were involved in a vitamin D supplementation study. Researchers found that the pregnant women with low vitamin D levels (defined in this study as below 20 ng/ml), increased the risk of passing HIV to their babies. HIV positive nursing mothers who were deficient in vitamin D were also more likely to pass HIV to their children. Higher mortality rates were also found for children born to mothers who were deficient in vitamin D. Researchers in this study suggest that vitamin D supplementation could be a simple and cost effective way to prevent HIV transmission from mothers to children and help save lives.

Babies and Children Need Vitamin D Too

You may be concerned about giving vitamin D supplements to your children. Many studies show that vitamin D helps to prevent many more diseases than rickets in children. Asthma, bronchitis, the common cold, swine flu and depression are some of the conditions which affect children and which vitamin D helps to prevent and control. New studies recommend that children be given vitamin D dosages that are higher than the current RDA. One study found that children in Finland had eighty percent less chance of developing type 1 diabetes when they were given 2,000 IU of vitamin D daily. Babies who are given vitamin D supplements have fewer colds. Equally important, ensuring that children's vitamin D levels are adequate during the early years can reduce the risk of many chronic and degenerative diseases during later years. Many adult diseases are associated with vitamin D deficiency in childhood.

All children, but especially black children, should be encouraged to spend time in the sun each day. Dark-skinned children have natural built-in sun block in their skin so they do not require sunscreen for protection in the same way that light-skinned children do. In addition to having a natural sun block which makes sunscreen largely unnecessary for dark-skinned children, using sunscreen might pose health dangers because of toxic chemicals that have been found in many sunscreen products. The *Environmental Working Group* reports that many sunscreen products may not provide the protection promised and that about half of the 500 most popular sunscreen products may be dangerous to your health. Chemicals in these sunscreen products may stimulate cancer growth. Children who are exposed to the dangerous chemicals in sunscreen products may be in even greater danger. Remember that if you live in a high latitude, sunlight-poor region, you will not get much vitamin D from the sun in the months between November and March. However, regardless of the time of year, when enough time cannot be spent in the sun, it is vital that you supplement your children with vitamin D. You should monitor your child's vitamin D levels in the same way you monitor your own. Have your child tested in order to determine blood vitamin D levels and follow up with advice from medical personnel regarding adequate vitamin D supplementation.

Vitamin D Needs of Breastfed Children

Although incomparably rich in vital nutrients necessary for young children's healthy growth and development, human milk is generally a poor source of vitamin D and black women, known to be critically deficient in vitamin D, provide their nursing infants with even less vitamin D from breast milk. Medical practitioners recommend that nursing mothers take 4,000 IU to 6,000 IU of vitamin D each day and that breastfed children be supplemented with vitamin D. Vitamin D supplements are available as drops, which can be conveniently given to infants.

It is of extreme importance that mothers be aware of the likelihood of vitamin D deficiency in their young children. Experts note that an infant who has head sweats at nights may be deficient in vitamin D. However, signs of vitamin D insufficiency may not always be visible. Nursing mothers and breastfed children should therefore be tested for vitamin D sufficiency. It bears repeating that vitamin D deficiency in infancy is linked to wide ranging health problems later in life, including auto immune diseases, cancer, diabetes, and nervous disorders.

Autism – Higher Incidence in Black Children

Autism is very common in the United States of America and has been found to be more prevalent among children whose mothers are black. Many experts believe that vitamin D deficiency plays a big role in the current high level of autism in the United States. *The Vitamin D Council* informs us that the theory that autism is caused from vitamin D deficiency in pregnancy is still only a theory. However, *The Council* points out that there is a plausible connection between autism and vitamin D deficiency due to significantly decreased sunlight exposure over the last 20 years. The last twenty years of decreased exposure to sunlight has also seen an exponential increase in autism cases.

The autism epidemic is more dire for darkly pigmented people who live in high latitude regions such as northern U.S., Canada, Britain, and other European countries. Children of Caribbean immigrants in Britain suffer higher rates of autism. Children born to other black immigrants in Europe suffer similarly high rates of autism. Researchers have found that the incidence of autism and related illnesses is three to four times higher among Somali immigrants living in Stockholm, Sweden. Researchers tell us that autism is so new to the Somali that these immigrants call autism the Swedish disease. In one study, Somali mothers were tested for vitamin D status, six years after they gave birth. The tests showed that mothers of autistic children had lower vitamin D levels than mothers of non-autistic children. Based on the effect of mother's vitamin D level on the unborn child, vitamin D experts advise that pregnant mothers take 5,000 IU of vitamin D every day. Darkly pigmented mothers may need more than this amount because of the barrier that the high melanin content of their skin presents to producing adequate vitamin D from sunlight.

Chapter 10

How Much Vitamin D Is Enough?

Many factors help to determine how much vitamin D your body needs and how much you should take. It is best to have your vitamin D level tested and to be guided by a doctor or other medical professional who is aware of the recent scientific research about vitamin D needs of the general population, and the health dilemma that dark-skinned people have been facing as a result of being so critically deficient in vitamin D. Given the health dangers of low vitamin D production due to highly melanized skin and inadequate sun exposure, it is vitally important that people with dark skin pigmentation supplement their diets with vitamin D. Previous chapters explain how conditions such as diseases, age, geographical location and sun exposure may affect your vitamin D needs. This chapter will give you suggestions about dosages and how factors such as prescription and over the counter medications may affect your vitamin D levels.

Dosages and Blood Level Measures

Supplementation of 5,000 IU daily of vitamin D is the amount that scientists claim the average person needs to prevent and control diseases. According to recent research, daily dosage of vitamin D may be suitable in the range of 5,000 to 6,000 IU for healthy dark pigmented adults. If you are extremely deficient or you suffer from chronic diseases such as cancer or diabetes you may need to take dosages higher than 6, 000 IU of vitamin D per day. The not-for-profit *Vitamin D Council* recommends that healthy children up to 2 years get 1,000 IU of vitamin D per day, healthy children 2 years and above get 2,000 per day and adolescents and adults who are healthy take 5,000 IU per day. Since dark pigmented children, adolescents and adults produce less vitamin D from the sun, one may imagine that their recommended daily dosage would need to be more than this.

You may try to get higher dosage amounts from reputable companies that have D3 supplements supplying 2,000 IU to 5,000 IU in capsule or in liquid form. Be aware that the vitamin D content that is stated on many vitamin D supplements may be misleading. A group of multiple sclerosis centers carried out a test on 10 different brands of vitamin D and found that the stated amounts were incorrect. All 10 brands were purchased at health food stores and online. These brands of vitamin D had actual dosages that were only about one-third of what the labels on the bottles stated. Many doctors and nutritionists supply vitamin D and other products directly to their clients because many supplements sold in health food stores, pharmacies and supermarkets can be very compromised.

Monitoring Your Blood Vitamin D Levels

It is important to monitor your blood vitamin D levels. Some researchers have found that an adult's body uses about 3,000 IU to 5,000 IU of vitamin D per day and will store excess vitamin D for about 6 months, before being replenished. However, you should make sure to have your blood vitamin D level tested. This will indicate whether you may need to take more than the recommended 5,000 IU per day. Experts now believe that adequate blood measurements are between 50 and 75 ng/ml (nanograms per milliliter). Blood level readings below 30 ng/ml indicate that you do not have sufficient vitamin D in your blood, and a reading below 20 ng/ml means that you are critically deficient in vitamin D. If your level is in excess of 100 ng/ml your body has excess vitamin D and 150 ng/ml indicates an intoxication point for vitamin D. See the chart below for an easy reference guide. You should bear in mind that recent scientific literature shows that supplementation with 1,000 IU per day is not likely to raise your level of vitamin D above 30 ng/ml. A daily dosage of 1,000 IU will not raise the blood vitamin D level of a dark pigmented person who is deficient in vitamin D to any point that is close to 30 ng/ml. Consequently, increased supplementation may be necessary.

The need for vitamin D is so great and its disease preventing ability so profound that a few companies are now making vitamin D supplements in dosages of 10,000 IU. However, before taking such a high dosage you should have your blood tested in order to determine whether you have sufficient vitamin D. Persons very deficient in vitamin D are sometimes required to supplement with vitamin D in weekly dosages as high as 50,000 IU. Doctors may recommend that patients take 50,000 IU of vitamin D for about eight weeks, followed by smaller dosages of 5,000 IU or less on a daily basis. This may be compared with the current United States recommended daily allowance (RDA) of 600 IU. Experts think that the U.S. RDA for vitamin D is much too low to maintain your health. The vitamin D content of milk, orange juice and boxed cereals is based on this very low RDA. You should not depend on vitamin D fortified foods to supply the amount of vitamin D that you need to sustain optimal health.

Health Effects of Vitamin D Blood Levels in ng/ml*

Health Effects	Vitamin D Level
Deficiency	Less than 20
Insufficiency	20 – 32
Sufficiency	32 – 75
Healthier Range	75-100
Excess	Higher than 100
Intoxication	Higher than 150

*ng/ml – nanograms per milliliter

Health Effects of Vitamin D Blood Levels in nmol/L*

Health Effects	Vitamin D Level
Deficiency	Less than 50
Insufficiency	50-80
Sufficiency	80-250
Healthier Range	185-250
Excess	Higher than 250
Intoxication	Higher than 325

* nmol/L – nanomoles per liter

How Medication May Affect
Your Vitamin D Levels

One of the frequent questions asked at my health care workshops has to do with how vitamin D interacts with prescription drugs. Research shows that there are usually no adverse reactions when you take vitamin D while taking prescription drugs. However, there are many medications that may reduce or deplete your vitamin levels. Cancer drugs, high blood pressure medication and others are some of the treatments that may lower the amount of vitamin D in your body, causing you to need more vitamin D.

Vitamin D is a natural substance that is provided abundantly and freely. The elements that go together to form vitamin D are part of the universal realm of life-sustaining substances. This helps to explain why vitamin D does not seem to have dangerous reactions with substances that can be ingested as food or medication. Like the whole foods we eat, vitamin D sustains health and life.

Prescription Drugs and Herbal Remedies
That May Reduce Your Vitamin D Levels

Some Cholesterol Drugs can cause your body to absorb less vitamin D from your supplement. If you must take a cholesterol drug, make sure that you take your vitamin D supplement two to four hours after you take this prescription medication.

High Blood Pressure Drugs can cause you to need more vitamin D. When you take water pills (diuretics) to reduce high blood pressure, your body may become more deficient in magnesium, calcium, potassium and vitamin D. Frequent urination causes excessive amounts of vitamin D and other nutrients to be excreted from your body.

Obesity-related Drugs decrease the absorption of dietary fats as well as vitamin D. Persons taking obesity-related drugs should keep their vitamin D intake at the upper recommended level. Bear in mind also, that obesity reduces the absorption of vitamin D, because fat cells in the body sequester vitamin D making the vitamin less available to cells of your body.

Depression and Anti-seizure Drugs that are used to treat depression and epilepsy destroy vitamin D. Patients who are on these medications often develop pain in their muscles and bones because they become deficient in vitamin D. This is considered to be one of the reasons why persons with depression and other forms of mental illnesses, often have physical disabilities. Medical personnel recommend that patients on seizure or psychiatric medication be given higher doses of vitamin D while they are on psychiatric medications.

Drugs Used in Immunotherapy treatment for AIDS, Organ Transplant, etc. Drugs that are used for immunotherapy also destroy vitamin D. AIDS and other immuno-compromised patients are in great need of vitamin D but medication for their illnesses lowers the amount of vitamin D available from vitamin D supplements. These patients should have their doctors prescribe appropriate amounts of vitamin D at higher levels. No one, and especially immuno-compromised patients, should depend on the small amount of vitamin D that is found in multivitamins.

Asthma Medication. The use of asthma medication, inhaled or taken orally, seems to reduce vitamin D in the body and increases the need to take vitamin D supplements.

Herbal Remedies. Herbs such as St. John's Wort can make less vitamin D available to your body. It is recommended that your vitamin D dosage be at increased levels.

Other Factors That May Reduce Your Vitamin D Levels

Smoking. Smoking has a deleterious effect on your body's ability to absorb and make use of vitamin D and calcium. Smoking may also reduce your bone mineral density and render you susceptible to musculoskeletal disorders such as osteoporosis.

Fat substitutes in "no-fat" chips interfere with the absorption of vitamin D. Fat free brands of traditional high-fat foods, such as potato chips, contain vitamin D inhibiting substances.

Deficiencies related to malfunctions in the body. Some illnesses can contribute to vitamin D deficiency. If you have a medical complaint, be sure to get advice from your physician about increasing your vitamin D dosage.

Vitamin D for Everyone

Vitamin D is so essential to life that everyone needs to be optimized with it. The current RDA of 600 IU may not prevent vitamin D deficiency. Most of the foods we eat today do not have enough vitamin D to maintain optimum vitamin D levels and multivitamins do not supply enough vitamin D to keep your body optimized. The Recommended Daily Allowance (RDA) for nutrients including vitamin D is set for the general population, not for special needs groups or for people with illnesses. Many blacks have unique vitamin D requirements because of the dark pigmentation of their skin.

It is not too early to take vitamin D to prevent illnesses; neither is it too late to optimize vitamin D levels to treat health problems. Studies show that vitamin D can alleviate common health problems that may show up in all age groups. We have heard of babies having weak bones or rickets and adults having muscle and bone pain or osteomalacia. These conditions develop over a short period of time and can usually be similarly reversed over a short period of time when adequate vitamin D is taken and calcium and magnesium levels are optimal. High melanin concentration in the skin of many blacks causes them to be deficient in vitamin D oftentimes starting before birth and continuing for their entire lives. Long-term vitamin D deficiency causes many of the chronic diseases that disproportionately affect blacks. It is therefore imperative that dark-skinned people of all ages and ancestries ensure that their vitamin D levels are optimized.

Your body will make more effective use of vitamin D when you eat healthy foods and exercise. The following chapters present important exercise and healthy eating tips and healthy recipes. Go to www.healthieryounutrition.com for more healthy eating tips and recipes.

PART TWO

Preventing Diseases and Healing the Body with Exercise and Healthy Foods

Chapter 11

Exercise – An Essential Health Factor

You need to move your body parts or you lose them. There really is no way to get around this absolutely crucial factor in your health. One report about hospital patients during World War II bears this out quite well. There were not enough beds so many of the patients who were hospitalized during WWII had to do without beds. To the surprise of medical personnel, patients who had no beds experienced faster wound healing, had less infection rates, and got earlier discharge from the hospital. This section on exercise is meant to remind you of the benefits of exercise.

The benefits of regular exercise cannot be overstated. Among other things, exercise helps to reduce stress, improves your cardiovascular system, helps to transport nutrients from the foods you eat into your cells, helps to oxygenate your cells, enhances the proper functioning of your digestive system, helps maintain proper hormone regulation, and facilitates the transport of waste products from your body. Regular, effective exercise gives you greater bone mass and muscle strength, better coordination and balance, and stronger heart and lung muscles. Exercise also contributes to good emotional health. You may find that you are calmer, more relaxed, and enjoy more restful sleep when you exercise.

Exercise and Vitamin D

Perhaps most important, is the finding that exercise and vitamin D share a wonderful reciprocal relationship. Exercise increases your vitamin D levels while having adequate vitamin D levels in turn helps you to optimize the benefits you get from exercising. You may recall from our discussion in chapter 5 that obesity inhibits the production of vitamin D as fat cells sequester vitamin D, preventing it from being properly used by the body. Fat loss, promoted by fat burning exercise, helps to free the storage of vitamin D from fat cells in the body thereby making it more available for use. In particular, muscle-building exercise has been associated with increased levels of vitamin D. This finding holds great significance for everyone, especially middle-aged and elderly persons who stand to benefit tremendously from weight bearing and muscle-building exercises.

Adequate vitamin D levels are associated with increased muscle strength. Vitamin D deficiency is associated with muscle weakness and increased susceptibility to falls and fractures in the elderly. Researchers have also found that vitamin D sufficiency in young women is associated with increased muscle mass and increased muscle strength. Given these findings, it seems plausible that having adequate vitamin D levels may increase the effectiveness of exercise as adequate vitamin D levels may contribute to muscle building and muscle strength.

Adequate vitamin D levels have also been found to increase your ability to breathe well. This holds much significance for increasing the effectiveness of exercise since adequate oxygen uptake by your lungs enhances oxygen circulation throughout your body as you exercise and consequently your endurance levels.

Exercise for Children

Children who regularly skip, run, jump, climb trees, and participate in organized physical activities also tend to be less moody and are less likely to be irritable and easily distracted. You may want to keep exercise fun for kids by going biking with your children, taking an exercise class with them, or by making jogging a family affair in the park. The website www.letsmove.gov

suggests how you may help children engage in physical activities each day.

Exercise for Middle-Aged and Elderly Persons

Activities such as walking, gardening, and yard work are great exercises for elderly persons. However, as mentioned earlier, middle aged and elderly persons should make weight-bearing exercises a regular part of their routine. Elderly people have more confident, upright gait, fewer falls and less bone fractures when they exercise regularly. Movement against gravity, especially weight bearing exercise, is good for bones and muscles. If you are a middle aged or elderly person and you haven't been exercising regularly, you should start slowly and gradually increase your effort at heavier weights as well as challenging aerobic activities. Regular stretching activities may also help to improve your flexibility.

Make Exercise Fun

Your exercise routine should be fun. Too many people fail to exercise or give up on exercising because they do not enjoy it. If you choose an exercise routine that you enjoy and find engaging you are more likely to stick with it. You may not even have to go to a gym. Listen to your body and find something you enjoy and which works for you.

Chapter 12

Tips for Selecting and Preparing Healthy Foods

The food you eat is the foundation of your health. Foods have disease preventing and healing qualities. Healthy eating has the potential to keep you in good health at every age and stage of life. Your genes influence your health but the foods you eat may have much greater effect on your health and well-being. More than 80 percent of diseases are nutrition related and recent studies show that a healthy diet can neutralize the effects of inherited tendency for diseases. You can minimize the effects of "bad genes" with good food and render "good genes" almost worthless with unhealthy eating. Family medical history is often used by doctors to assess disease conditions and make prognoses. However, more doctors should incorporate dietary habits into health assessments for their patients.

What is healthy eating? Which foods promote good health and help fight disease? Which ones make you susceptible to disease and ill-health? Below are tips on food selection and preparation, which should serve as useful guidelines for healthy eating.

Healthy Eating Tips

Eat Lots of:

1.

Whole, Real Foods: Eat a well balanced diet focusing on wholesome foods including fresh vegetables and fruits, grass-fed organic meats, good fats, soaked grains, and good quality water.

2.

Good Quality Water. Good quality water is essential to good health. Our bodies are mostly water because water is needed to carry out all the chemical processes in our bodies. Most bottled water is a waste of your hard earned money as many of them are not as pure or well filtered as their manufacturers claim. Your best bet for ensuring that you and your family are drinking good quality water daily is to make sure you have a high quality, reputable water filtration system in your home not only for your drinking water but also for the water you bathe in. You may visit www.healthieryounutrition.com for suggestions on good quality water filters.

3.

Organic Fruits and Vegetables. Organic fruits and vegetables supply our bodies with a lot of the water that our bodies need to maintain good health. They also supply more vitamins and minerals than their conventional counterparts. Non-organic fruits and vegetables are oftentimes laden with pesticides which have been associated with a host of diseases and are especially harmful to young children and pregnant women. Always try to get organic versions of thin-skinned produce as these fruits and vegetables are more susceptible to absorbing pesticides. Look for the USDA organic seal when shopping. The price look up code (PLU code) for organic produce usually has 5 digits beginning with the number 9.

The Environmental Working Group, a not-for-profit consumer advocacy group, published their most recent findings on tests done on levels of pesticides in common fruits and vegetables. According to the findings, you should always try to buy organic versions of these fruits and vegetables commonly referred to as the dirty dozen because of the high levels of pesticides often found in the non-organic versions: celery, peaches, strawberries, apples, blueberries, nectarines, bell peppers, spinach, cherries, kale, collard greens, potatoes, and imported grapes. You can get conventional versions of more thick skinned produce such as pineapple, mangoes, watermelon, and cantaloupe. Remember that washing pesticide-laden fruits and vegetables will not necessarily remove the contaminants as many of them are completely absorbed by the fruit or vegetable and not just found on the skin. You can download the complete shopper's guide to pesticides at http://www.foodnews.org/walletguide.php. Also remember that eating locally grown, pesticide free produce is always advisable. Besides supporting local farmers and your local economy, locally grown produce tends to be fresher than produce which has to travel long distances before you purchase them in a store. For reputable local producers in your area, go to www.localharvest.org.

4.

Good Quality Fats. Not all fats are bad for you. Good fats, especially omega-3 essential fatty acids (omega-3 EFAs) are vital for good health. Low levels of omega-3 have been associated with cancer, heart disease, hypertension, diabetes, obesity, mental illness such as depression, schizophrenia, Alzheimer's, attention deficit disorder, and a host of other chronic diseases. Food sources rich in omega-3 include fatty fish such as wild salmon. Supplementing with omega-3 fish oils is a good idea but remember that some fish oils do not have high omega-3 content while other fish oils may have come from fish exposed to dangerous industrial wastes such as PCBs. You may visit www. healthieryounutrition.com for recommendations for reputable brands of fish oil.

Other sources of good fats include coconut oil and butter from grass-fed cattle. Lauric acid, the main fatty acid from coconut oil, converts to monolaurin in the body which plays an especially important role in good health as it has powerful antiviral, antibacterial, and antifungal properties. Lauric acid has been shown to have broad-spectrum effectiveness against viruses such as HIV, influenza, herpes, pathogenic bacteria such as helicobacter pylori, a common culprit in stomach disorders, and yeast such as candida albicans.

5.

Organic, Grass Fed Meats come from animals that feed freely on pastures. Organic, pastured meats are healthier for you for a number of reasons. They provide you with a significantly higher percentage of good fats than animals which are fed grains such as corn and soy, and raised in conventional factory, feed lot conditions. Also, meat from pastured animals is rich in omega-3 EFAs. In addition, they are richer in antioxidants, especially vitamin E, and they do not have drugs such as antibiotics and growth hormones. Grass fed beef is especially rich in an essential fatty acid known as conjugated linoleic acid, CLA, which has broad spectrum health promoting properties. High levels of CLA in the diet have been shown to help mitigate cancer, high blood pressure, osteoporosis, and inflammation. CLA has also been shown to help lower body fat. Eating lots of fresh, organic dark green leafy vegetables with your meats may reduce the acid forming potential of meat. The website www.eatwild.com lists reputable providers of grass fed meats.

6.

Dairy products from pastured animals. It should come as no surprise that eggs, butter, and milk from pastured animals are much better for you than those from conventionally raised animals. For example, free range eggs from chickens that are allowed to range freely and forage all day, have far more nutrients than eggs from conventionally raised chickens typically fed diets of corn and soy. The not for profit, Cornucopia Institute, recently released findings from a comprehensive study of egg producers in which it rated suppliers of factory farm mass produced eggs versus authentic free range eggs. You can find the report at http://www.cornucopia.org/2010/09/organic-egg-report-and-scorecard/. You can also go to www.eatwild.com and www.local

harvest.org for reputable providers of dairy products from pastured animals.

7.

Breakfast. Although it may be tempting and convenient to do so, you should not skimp on breakfast or take shortcuts with your breakfast. Eating a healthy breakfast is essential to your good health. Breakfast replenishes your blood sugar levels and fuels you with energy for the day. Studies have shown that eating a healthy breakfast promotes a healthy body mass index (BMI). Further, people who eat breakfast are less likely to develop diabetes and high blood pressure than people who don't. A healthy breakfast is especially important for growing children. Children who eat a high quality breakfast have better attention span, mood, memory, and tend to perform better academically and athletically than those who don't. Your breakfast should be a combination of high quality proteins, good fats, vegetables, and fruits. Go to www.healthieryounutrition.com for free breakfast recipes.

8.

Crucifers. Cruciferous vegetables or crucifers such as broccoli, Brussels sprouts, kale, and collard greens are powerful health promoters. Clinical trials show that crucifers possess anticancer properties and these foods can protect your body against substances such as histone deacetylases (HDACs) - enzymes in your body that have the ability to alter good genes. You have good genes that help to keep off diseases, but HDACs can lower the activity of good genes that ward off diseases such as cancer. Crucifers such as cabbage, broccoli, Brussels sprouts and collard greens contain substances that inhibit the action of histone deacetylases (HDACs). HDAC inhibitors in cruciferous vegetables help to prevent diseases such as cancers.

9.

Alliaceae – Members of the Onion Family. Like *crucifers* mentioned above, *alliaceae* contain cancer fighting substances known as organosulfur compounds. These sulfur compounds which may help to prevent cancer, include sulforaphane in broccoli, indole-3-carbinol in cabbage, and at least 8 organosulfur compounds in the onion and garlic species. Organosulfur compounds in foods from the cabbage and onion families may stop the action of dangerous HDACs in your body and protect you from diseases such as cancers.

10.

Flavonoids and Carotenoids. Flavonoids are chemical substances found in fruits and vegetables. They act as natural antioxidants and anti-inflammatory agents and offer powerful protection against a host of chronic diseases. Carotenoids are the substances which give fruits and vegetables their yellow and orange colors. Eat a diverse array of fresh vegetables and fruits and you will have the disease fighting protection of flavonoids and carotenoids. If you are concerned about not having the time to make sure you meet your daily nutritional requirements for antioxidant rich fruits and vegetables you should consider juicing. Juicing is an excellent way to ensure you are meeting your daily nutritional needs of antioxidant rich fruits and vegetables. Visit www.healthieryounutrition.com for recommended juicers.

11.

Nuts. Nuts may protect your heart. The overall risk for heart disease appears to be lower in people who ate nuts one or more times per week. Nuts are high in vitamin E, magnesium and potassium, and are good suppliers of good fats. Walnuts are especially high in the omega-3 fat, alpha-linoleic acid (ALA). ALA has been shown to support healthy heart rhythm and reduce sudden death from heart attacks in people who previously suffered heart attacks. Caution should however be exercised in eating nuts to supply most of your omega-3 needs. ALA from plant sources do not convert to the longer chain omega-3s (EPA and

DHA) that come from fish oils. You may also need to avoid eating large amounts of nuts when you are overweight or diabetic.

Completely Avoid or Extremely Limit Your Consumption of:

1.

Sugar. Excessive consumption of sugar severely compromises your immune system and is a major contributor to chronic health problems including cancer and obesity. High fructose corn syrup is perhaps the most widely consumed form of sugar and it is also one of the most dangerous forms of sugar. High fructose corn syrup is found in most processed foods we eat today. You need to read supermarket food labels very carefully because high fructose corn syrup is typically cleverly disguised under many labels such as corn syrup, fruit fructose, glucose syrup, crystalline fructose, chicory, and tapioca syrup. If you try to stick with wholesome unprocessed foods you will significantly limit your intake of sugar and especially high fructose sugar.

2.

Genetically Modified Foods. Avoiding genetically modified foods is becoming increasingly difficult to do since so many forms of genetically modified foods abound in cleverly disguised forms in much of the foods we eat today. Genetically modified foods have been associated with hormonal disruption and imbalance, most notably disruption of the hormone insulin. Corn and soy are two of the most common foods that are typically genetically engineered. Your best bet for avoiding genetically modified foods is to stick with wholesome, unprocessed, and organic foods. This will greatly minimize the amount of genetically modified foods you eat. For more information on how to avoid genetically modified foods, download the non-gmo food shopping guide for free at http://www.nongmoshoppingguide.com.

3.

Soy. In addition to oftentimes being genetically modified, soy foods can disrupt endocrine function and can stimulate the growth of cancer cells. Eating soy foods can also contribute to hypothyroidism and result in weight gain and fatigue. Soy foods contain high concentrations of brain toxins such as fluoride and glutamate and have been linked to Parkinson's disease. Exceptions to this are organic fermented soy foods like natto and tempeh.

4.

Boxed Cereals. Most boxed cereals are made by a process known as extrusion which destroys many nutrients in grains and turns some food substances toxic. The extrusion process effectively destroys the fatty acids and amino acids found in grains. Boxed cereals sold in health food stores are typically made by the same extrusion process. The best way to have grains for cereal is to soak them overnight and make old-fashioned porridge. Soaking grains helps to reduce their phytic acid content and consequently increases their digestibility and absorption. Phytic acid in grains inhibits absorption of vital minerals such as calcium, magnesium, copper, iron, and zinc. Soaking also helps to make gluten, which is difficult to digest, more digestible.

5.

Fat-Free Snacks. Fat-free snacks may result in more harm than good to your health. Fat substitutes used in potato and other chips may prevent vitamin D from being absorbed into your body. This contradicts your purpose for choosing fat free foods because vitamin D which helps to prevent obesity is being blocked. It is interesting to note that olestra, a fat substitute in fat-free chips, has been banned in some countries.

6.

Excessive alcohol. Alcohol uses up your important B vitamins and a deficiency of B vitamins can cause you to become depressed. When your body is deficient in the B complex group of vitamins you become susceptible to many illnesses.

7.

Food Additives. Food additives are used to enhance the flavor and color of processed foods and extend their shelf life. Studies have shown that many of the food additives being used in processed foods are associated with chronic diseases including cancer, neurological disturbances, and hormonal imbalance. Be sure to read product labels carefully. Some of the most commonly used ones include artificial colorings, aspartame-artificial sweetener, sodium nitrite, BHA, BHT, monosodium glutamate (MSG), sodium benzoate, fructose, and high fructose corn syrup. Eating whole, unprocessed foods is the best way to avoid harmful food additives, which are found in most processed foods. The table below highlights some common food additives and the foods in which they are usually found.

Food Additive	Usually found in	Health Danger
Monosodium Glutamate (MSG)	Soups, bouillon cubes, soup noodles, barbecue sauces, canned foods, potato chips, tortilla chips, seasoning mixtures, frozen food, and many restaurant foods.	Destroys brain cells, contributes to a host of chronic diseases, including diabetes, obesity, Alzheimer's, and cancer. MSG also causes migraine headaches and depression.

High Fructose Corn Syrup	Most processed foods including breads, cereals, soft drinks, sauces, salad dress-ings, popcorn	May cause diabetes, high blood pressure, high cholesterol, obesity, heart disease and depression and aggressiveness in children.
Sodium nitrate/nitrite	Luncheon meats, ham, hot dogs, bacon	Has been associated with many types of cancer.
Sodium Benzoate	Soft drinks, fruit juices, energy drinks	Has been shown to cause hyper-activity and reduced attention span.
Aspartame	Diet sodas, other sodas	May worsen diabetes, and cause high blood pressure, heart disease, and depression.
Artificial food colors	Drinks, baked foods, candy	Have been shown to cause hyper-activity and low IQ in children.

8.

Mercury Laden Fish. Many farm raised fish are notoriously high in mercury, a highly toxic chemical which can cause damage to your brain and other organs in your body. Wild caught fish is generally not as toxic as farm-raised fish. Wild caught oily fish such as salmon is especially good for you due to its high omega 3 content. Visit www.seafoodwatch.org for detailed information on seafood recommendations.

9.

Sodas. Sodas are laden with sugar, especially high fructose corn syrup, and other additives that are extremely damaging to your health. Studies have shown that sodas, diet and regular, are associated with diabetes, high blood pressure, obesity, attention deficit disorder, and a host of other illnesses.

10.

Avoid Bisphenol-A (BPA) and most Canned Foods. Almost all canned products, including those labeled organic, are lined with BPA, a dangerous chemical that has been associated with cancer and reproductive abnormalities. Some manufacturers are making BPA free cans--be sure to check the label or do some investigating before buying. If you try to eat mainly fresh, unprocessed foods you will significantly limit your exposure to BPA.

Babies are also in danger because 95 percent of all baby bottles in the USA are made with BPA which can compromise healthy, normal development in babies. Canada and countries in the European Union have banned the use of BPA in baby bottles. In September 2010, Canada, the first country to officially ban BPA in baby bottles, declared BPA a toxic substance. The U.S.A. has not banned the use of BPA. However, the United States Food and Drug Administration has changed its position about BPA by voicing concern about the effects of BPA on the brain, behavior, and sex organs of unborn babies and young children.

Food Preparation Tips

1.

Steam vegetables lightly. If you need to cook vegetables it is best to steam them lightly and not for very long. Light steaming will preserve the valuable vitamins and minerals and some of the enzymes in vegetables. A vegetable steamer is an important and very useful piece of equipment to have in your kitchen.

2.

Use whole foods for creative toppings. Be creative with your use of whole foods for toppings. For example, sprinkle ground flaxseed or wheat bran on your porridge or yogurt. These are good for your heart, nerves, and mood.

3.

Help to Prevent Cancer by Marinating Meat in Herbs. Season your meat by soaking it in a marinade made from herbs and spices such as thyme, garlic, green onions, rosemary, ginger, oregano, basil and sage. When you cook beef, fish, pork or poultry at high temperatures amino acids in these foods form cancer-causing compounds called heterocyclic amines (HCAs). *The Journal of Food Science* reports that HCA levels in steak drop by as much as 88 percent when steak is marinated in seasonings made from different herbs and spices before cooking. Each herb or spice has its unique health benefits therefore a mixture of herbs and spices will enhance potency and increase health benefits. *The Journal of Medicinal Foods* lists herbs and spices that rank highest for preventing premature aging and diseases. Some of the major herbs and spices listed are cloves, cinnamon, Jamaican allspice or pimento, oregano, marjoram, sage, thyme and Italian spice mixture.

4.

Reduce Time Spent in the Kitchen and Still Eat Well. If possible, set aside some time shortly after you shop for groceries. Wash your meats, cut into desired pieces according to the meals you will prepare for the week. Next, pound your green herbs and spices using a pestle and mortar and place meats in different marinade mixtures of pounded herbs. Divide meats into daily portions, place in freezer bags and freeze. When you want to prepare a meal, simply grab a bag from the freezer. You may prefer to cook all your meats for the week at the same time by cooking big portions and freezing in smaller quantities that you and your family can have for meals throughout the week. Precut your vegetables and place them in freezer bags. When you are ready to have your meal, remove a bag or two of vegetables, empty them into a saucepan containing garlic and onion sautéed in coconut oil, or olive oil, steam lightly for a few minutes and you are ready to eat.

5.

Avoid Using Plastic Containers especially in the Microwave. Many plastic containers have bisphenol-A (BPA), a dangerous chemical which leaches into food or liquids. Repeated exposure to BPA has been associated with increased cancer risk and some experts believe it may also be linked to reproductive abnormalities. Try to use glass or stainless steel containers instead – especially for warm or hot foods.

Important Supplements

The standard American diet typically consists of foods that have lost a high percentage of nutrients due to processing. The United States Food and Drug Administration (FDA) reports that the average American diet may have less than 80 percent of the Recommended Daily Allowance (RDA) of many essential nutrients. Nutrient deficiency is worsened when you are exposed to stress, when you take prescription medication, and when your body is exposed to toxins from the environment. These conditions induce deficiency of food nutrients because important nutrients that would normally be used to nourish your body are instead used to regulate stress hormones and to detoxify chemicals that are absorbed by your body. In addition to a good multivitamin and a daily dosage of vitamin D, you may need to supplement with the following:

1. **Vitamin B12.** Vitamin B12 helps your energy, mood, mental clarity, concentration, memory, and overall immune function. Unfortunately, you may be deficient in B12 if you take medication, or you are over 50 years of age. A diet that is low in B12 may also cause you to be anemic. Vitamin B12 deficiency is linked to pernicious

anemia. There is no need to worry about overdosing on your daily dosage of B12 because this vitamin is not stored in your body for long periods of time. You therefore need B12 from foods or supplements daily.

2. **Vitamin C.** When taken regularly, this vitamin detoxifies the body and strengthens the immune system. Everyone needs this vitamin but if you are 50 years or above this nutrient is of paramount importance to you, and you may need to take it daily.

3. **Omega-3**. Omega 3 essential fatty acids, especially eicosapentaenoic acid (EPA) and docosahexaenoic acid (DHA) have broad spectrum beneficial effects on the entire body. EPA and DHA play an important role in the prevention of many diseases and disorders including cancer, depression, heart disease, diabetes, and arthritis.

4. **Calcium and magnesium**. Calcium and magnesium are minerals which work as important co-factors of vitamin D. They are both crucial for optimum heart health and play a vital role in the prevention of high blood pressure and other diseases.

5. **Vitamin K2.** The K2 form of vitamin K has recently been found to be extremely beneficial in helping to prevent heart disease. Without enough vitamin K2, calcium which you absorb with the help of vitamin D, accumulates in your coronary arteries which could eventually lead to heart disease. It is extremely important that you consume K2 rich foods such as organic natto and cheese from grass-fed animals to optimize your intake. If eating these foods isn't feasible then you should take a good quality K2 supplement.

6. **CoenzymeQ10 and Ubiquinol**. Coenzyme Q10 (CoQ10) and ubiquinol are powerful nutrients which your body needs more of as you age. Your body typically converts

CoQ10 to ubiquinol, but this ability diminishes as you get older. These powerful nutrients carry out a host of important functions in your body such as helping your cells to produce energy, protecting your heart, and boosting your immunity.

7. **Probiotics.** The seat of your immunity resides is in your digestive tract. Beneficial bacteria in probiotics help to improve digestion and gut issues and provide significant boost to your digestive function and overall health.

You may find suggestions for reputable providers of these supplements at www.healthieryounutrition.com.

Chapter 13

Fighting Inflammation with Anti-Inflammatory Foods

Inflammation is at the root of nearly every chronic health problem. Inflammation is the process by which your body tries to protect and repair itself from damage caused by environmental toxins, emotional stress, unhealthy foods, and physical injuries. Inflammation is beneficial to your body when your injured cells and tissues heal quickly. However, prolonged inflammation can create serious damage to your body. Many inflammatory diseases such as cancer, heart disease, diabetes, and Alzheimer's are diagnosed many years after the onset of inflammation in the body. The good news is that together with vitamin D and other important nutrients, anti-inflammatory foods can significantly reduce inflammation in your body and your risk of getting high blood pressure, heart disease, diabetes, strokes, cancers, and a host of other chronic diseases.

Anti-Inflammatory Foods

When it comes to inflammation and disease prevention, some foods are better than others. Your health will be greatly enhanced when you eat a wide variety of anti-inflammatory herbs, spices, vegetables, fruits, meats, and nuts. Be adventurous in selecting and mixing foods from different categories, colors, and textures. The tables below outline some major anti-inflammatory herbs, spices, vegetables, fruits, meats, and nuts and their nutritional benefits.

Herbs and Spices	Health Benefits
Cinnamon	Cinnamon regulates blood sugar, lowers bad cholesterol, helps prevent yeast infections, reduces growth of some cancer cells, and works as an anti-clotting factor in the blood. One half teaspoon of cinnamon powder per day may help control blood glucose.
Cloves	Cloves relieve pain and may help prevent stomach and colon cancer when used routinely in very small amounts. Cloves have one of the highest antioxidant activity of any food source.
Curcumin (turmeric)	Curcumin is a powerful anti-inflammatory food. It reduces damage from colitis, relieves rheumatoid arthritis, reduces damage of lungs and pancreas by cystic fibrosis, protects the cells of the colon and retards growth of cancer cells. It improves liver function, can stimulate healing of wounds, and provides brain protection.
Onion, Leeks, Shallots, Scallion	Support healthy blood flow, regulate heart function, and help prevent cancer.
Chili peppers	Chili peppers help prevent heart disease and cancer.
Ginger	Ginger has anti-inflammatory compounds that are said to relieve rheumatoid arthritis, gastrointestinal pain, and protect against cancer.
Garlic	Garlic is a powerful antioxidant. It is antiviral, antibacterial, and antifungal. Garlic lowers total cholesterol and lowers high blood pressure. Allicin found in garlic is a cancer preventive agent.

Vegetables and Fruits	Health Benefits
Dark Green Leafy Vegetables such as kale, collard greens, turnip greens, romaine lettuce, Swiss chard, bok choy, spinach, and others	Darker greens are nutrition power-houses loaded with essential vitamins and minerals that help to cleanse your blood. Have them cooked and uncooked to help to normalize blood pressure and reduce your risk of cancers, heart disease, strokes, diabetes and other diseases.
Brightly colored vegetables and fruits such as carrots, kabocha squash (pumpkin), sweet potatoes, mangoes, tomatoes, watermelon, and berries.	Brightly colored fruits and vegetables fight free radicals and boost immunity by lowering bad cholesterol, normalizing blood pressure, and supporting healthy vision.
Cabbage, Broccoli, Cauliflower and other Crucifers	These are immune system boosters that among other things prevent and fight cancers, lower risk of cataracts and heart disease.
Aloe vera	Aloe vera has anti-viral and anti-bacterial properties. It is an excellent vegetarian food because Aloe vera is the only known plant source of vitamin B12, a vitamin found in animal protein sources.
Okra	Okra is rich in vitamins, calcium, and other minerals. It helps prevent anemia, supports proper nerve function, and strengthens the immune system.
Avocado	Avocado contains high potassium and B vitamins, and has beneficial effects on cholesterol and blood pressure.

Kiwi	Kiwi is high in vitamin C which strengthens the immune system and helps protect against diseases such as cancer, high blood pressure, heart disease, asthma, and macular degeneration.
Pineapple	Pineapple has vitamins, minerals and enzymes that help to regulate the digestive system, reduce inflammation, and contribute to healthy weight.
Lemons, oranges, and other citrus fruits	Oranges and other citrus fruits possess powerful flavanoids that slow cancer growth, and guard against heart attacks and strokes. Orange pulp has 10 times the vitamin C found in the juice. You get superior health benefits when you consume fresh oranges, or high pulp orange juice.
West Indian Cherry	West Indian Cherry has many nutrients and is one of the highest known sources of vitamin C. It boosts immunity, prevents infections, repairs tissues, and promotes colon health, lowers risk of cancers, heart disease and other degenerative diseases. It also helps maintain good vision.
Pumpkin	Pumpkin is rich in carotenoids and protects against many types of cancer.
Sorrel (Florida Cranberry or Roselle)	Sorrel contains powerful anti-oxidants that help to detoxify the body and protect against cancers and other diseases.

Meats and Nuts	Health Benefits
Wild Salmon	Wild salmon is a powerful anti-inflammatory food which provides a multitude of benefits. High in omega 3's, wild salmon prevents inflammation and lowers risks for cancers, high blood pressure, heart disease, depression, Alzheimer's, macular degeneration, obesity, and diabetes.
Hormone-free Chicken	Hormone-free chicken has high quality protein that helps to prevent bone and muscle loss. It is rich in selenium and B vitamins that provide important antioxidant protection.
Grass-fed Beef	Among its many benefits, grass-fed beef is especially rich in conjugated linoleic acid (CLA), a potent nutrient which has been shown to have broad spectrum preventive effect against many diseases including many types of cancers, cardiovascular disease, diabetes, and osteoporosis. Grass fed beef also has very high vitamin E and vitamin B content.
Nuts	Nuts contain health enhancing nutrients such as the antioxidant selenium that reduces dangerous free radicals and helps prevent cancer. Nuts supply omega-3 fats that contribute to heart and brain health, prevent gall stone formation and help to produce serotonin.

Recipes

The recipes in this section use whole foods that have outstanding anti-inflammatory health effects. Regular preparation and consumption of foods included in this chapter, will give you the opportunity to use your kitchen as a health laboratory. Eating whole foods that are anti-inflammatory will help you conquer diseases and maintain optimum health. Additional recipes are available at www.healthieryounutrition.com.

Aloe Vera

Health Benefits of Aloe Vera: Aloe vera strengthens the immune system, reduces inflammation, destroys tumor cells, regulates blood sugar in diabetics, lowers cholesterol, prevents and reduces ulcers, controls heartburn and acid reflux disease, heals skin burns, relieves joint pain, reduces acne and enhances skin health. Many aloe vera drinks sold in retail stores are very diluted and some contain almost no aloe vera. Some might appear thicker than others, but makers of aloe vera juice often add thickeners and lots of harmful preservatives. Additionally, aloe vera juices sold in stores might have been heated, and heating destroys some of the health benefits. Be sure to read labels carefully when purchasing aloe vera juices.

Aloe Vera Power Blend

Serves 2

2 tablespoons aloe vera gel from a fresh, washed leaf
1 cup fresh pineapple cubes
1 small piece of ginger (about 1 tablespoonful when peeled, washed and chopped)
papaya (about ½ lb, washed, seeded, peeled and cubed)
2 tablespoons coconut milk
1 cup orange juice
4 ice cubes

* * * *

Place all ingredients in a blender and blend at medium speed for about 2 minutes. Serve chilled.

Pumpkin

Health Benefits of Pumpkin: Pumpkin is one of the richest suppliers of carotenoids and offers protection against lung, colon, breast, prostate and cervical cancers. Carotenoids found in pumpkin also lower the risk of cataracts and macular degeneration.

Pumpkin Stir Fry

Serves 3.

1½ lbs. pumpkin (kabucha) - seeded, washed and diced in 1-inch cubes
1 cup water
3 cloves garlic- cleaned, washed and crushed
1 stalk scallion – cleaned, washed and crushed
2 tablespoons olive oil
Pinch of sea salt to taste

* * * *

1. Bring water to a boil and add salt to taste.
2. Add pumpkin to water in pot, cover and cook on medium heat for about 10 minutes.
3. Remove pumpkin from water.
4. Place garlic, scallion and olive oil in a small saucepan and sauté on medium heat for about 2 minutes.
5. Add pumpkin to sautéed mixture and stir gently.
6. Place pumpkin stir-fry mixture in serving casserole and serve warm.

Turmeric/ Curcumin

Health Benefits of Turmeric: Turmeric, the main ingredient in curry powder, reduces damage to intestinal walls by inflammatory bowel diseases such as colitis, relieves rheumatoid arthritis, reduces damage to lungs and pancreas by cystic fibrosis and helps to protect the cells of the colon. It also improves liver function and helps prevent memory loss in the elderly.

Curried Cauliflower

Serves 4

12 oz. cauliflower florets
2 teaspoon curry powder
1 medium red onion, chopped
1/8 teaspoon chopped red chili pepper
2 tablespoons unrefined olive oil or unrefined coconut oil
Pinch of salt

* * * *

1. Place oil, pepper, onion, and curry in a large skillet and sauté on medium heat stirring constantly for about 1 or 2 minutes.
2. Reduce flame and stir in 5 tablespoons water.
3. Add cauliflower and mix in.
4. Cover and steam for about 5 minutes, stirring occasionally until cauliflower is tender but firm.

Sorrel/Roselle

Sorrel or Florida Cranberry, also called roselle, comes from the flower of a species of Hibiscus plant. Sorrel contains flavonoids that prevent inflammation in the body. Sorrel is available in the fresh as well as dried form. The dried form of sorrel can be stored in a container for many months before it is used, but sorrel drink has a better flavor when it is produced from freshly cut flowers. Some studies have found that sorrel might have some preventive effect against cancer.

Sorrel Drink

Serves 4

1 cup dried sorrel
1 cube fresh ginger
1 medium stick cinnamon
5 cups water
Juice of 1 lemon

* * * *

1. Place cleaned dry sorrel in a small pot.
2. Crush ginger and add to sorrel.
3. Add cinnamon stick and 5 cups of water.

4. Cover pot and bring ingredients to boil.
5. Lower heat and simmer for about 2 minutes.
6. Turn off flame and allow ingredients in pot to seep for at least 5 hours or overnight.
7. Strain liquid and pour in glass jar.
8. Add juice from one lemon and sweeten to taste. Serve with ice.

Watermelon

Health Benefits of Watermelon: Watermelon is a great thirst quencher for many. But did you know that watermelon has a bountiful supply of nutrients that prevent inflammation and keep off diseases? According to one 2007 study published in the journal *Nutrition,* when you drink watermelon juice daily for several weeks you help to protect your body against prostate cancer, high blood pressure and abnormal insulin secretion.

Watermelon Refresher

Serves 3

¼ of a large watermelon seeded and cubed—about 5 cups
juice of 1 lemon—about 3 tbsps
8 ice cubes

* * * *

Place watermelon in a blender, and add juice of 1 lemon and 8 ice cubes. Blend at medium speed for about 2 minutes. Serve immediately.

Dark Green Leafy Vegetables

Health Benefits of Greens: Greens are anti-aging, anti-cancer and anti-diabetes. The darkest greens supply the greatest bounty of nutrients. Romaine lettuce, for example, has 8 times the vitamin A and 6 times the vitamin C content of iceberg lettuce. Dark green leafy vegetables also control blood pressure, maintain the heart, and enhance skin health.

Collard Greens Stir Fry

Serves 4

1 lb collard greens, cleaned, washed and chopped
½ red bell pepper seeded and diced

¼ cup water

pinch of sea-salt

1 medium onion, cleaned, washed, and chopped

6 cloves garlic, cleaned, washed, and crushed

3 tablespoon unrefined coconut oil or unrefined olive oil

* * * *

1. Heat oil on medium flame, add onion and garlic, and sauté for 3 minutes until onion is translucent.

2. Stir in collard greens and bell pepper and steam on low heat until tender. Greens should retain their bright green color when done.

Wild Caught Salmon

Health Benefits of Wild Salmon: Wild salmon is rich in omega-3 fatty acids which reduce the risk of heart disease and support healthy brain function. Frequent eating of wild salmon may also slow the growth of plaque in the arteries and prevent high blood pressure. To retain maximum health benefits have your salmon grilled, steamed, or baked. Frying destroys nutrients.

Wild Salmon on Bed of Cabbage

Serves 4

1 lb wild salmon

2 tablespoon coconut oil or olive oil

4 leaves green basil, crushed, or 1 teaspoon dried basil

1 sprig fresh thyme, crushed

4 cloves garlic, cleaned, washed and crushed

1 small onion, cleaned, washed and minced

¼ teaspoon sea salt

1 lb cabbage, washed and cut in wedges

4 tablespoons water

* * * *

1. Place oil, basil, thyme, garlic and onion in a skillet, mix in salt and sauté on medium heat for 1- 2 minutes.

2. Cut salmon in 3 or 4 pieces and smother all sides in sautéed mixture, gently turning and heating salmon for 5 minutes.

3. Place cabbage in a sauté pan, arrange salmon and seasoning on top of cabbage in pan, and add water.
4. Cover and cook on medium to low temperature for 5-8 minutes, until cabbage is tender.
5. Carefully lift salmon and cabbage and serve on warm plates.

Organic, Pastured Chicken

Health Benefits of Pastured Chicken: Pastured chicken, unlike conventionally produced chicken, comes from birds that were given constant access to rich vegetation, fresh air, and sunshine. You should be aware that many chickens and other forms of poultry labeled "free-range" were not given access to outdoor vegetation. Besides being far more flavorful than conventionally produced chicken, truly pastured organic chicken has high quality protein that helps to prevent bone and muscle loss, and B vitamins, selenium, zinc and other minerals that provide antioxidant and immune defense.

Caribbean Curried Chicken

Serves 6 to 8

1 pastured chicken – about 4 lbs, washed and cut in 10 to 12 pieces
3-4 tablespoons Jamaican curry powder
4 sprigs thyme, washed and leaves removed and crushed, to be used in cooking
1 large onion, chopped
2 stalks scallion, cleaned, washed and crushed
½ of one hot pepper, chopped
1 teaspoon ground black pepper
1 inch cube fresh ginger, washed, skinned and grated
1 teaspoon salt
2 tablespoons unrefined coconut or unrefined olive oil
1 large white potato, peeled washed and diced
1 large carrot, peeled washed and diced
1 cup water

* * * *

1. Place chicken in a large bowl.

2. Sprinkle on chicken curry powder, crushed thyme, chopped onion, crushed scallion, chopped pepper, black pepper, grated ginger, and salt.
3. Marinate chicken in seasoning mixture at least 1 hour.
4. Pour oil in a large skillet and heat over medium flame.
5. Add chicken with seasoning and sauté until chicken is thoroughly heated.
6. Add water and cook chicken for 30 minutes.
7. Add diced potatoes and carrots and cook for an additional 10 minutes.

Grass-fed Beef

> **Health Benefits of Grass Fed Beef:** One of the main benefits of grass fed beef is its very high conjugated linoleic acid (CLA) content. CLA, a nutrient found in the fat of animals that feed on green grass, has been found to be highly protective against cancer, high blood pressure, osteoporosis, and inflammation. CLA is also found in butterfat from grass fed cattle.

Peppered Steak

<u>Serves 5</u>

1 lb grass fed beef, round or flank, cleaned and cut in ¼ inch wide strips
3 tablespoons unrefined coconut oil or olive oil
3 large green bell peppers, washed, seeded and cut in ½ inch strips
1 medium onion, cleaned, washed and sliced
3 stalks celery, washed and diced – about 1 cup
1 lb tomatoes, washed and chopped
1 teaspoon arrowroot powder
¼ cup water
1 teaspoon sea salt
4 cloves crushed garlic
2 bay leaves

* * * *

1. Heat oil in a skillet over medium heat.
2. Add beef to oil and allow to brown lightly.
3. Remove beef from oil, set aside and reduce heat.
4. Place onion in oil and allow to sauté for 3 minutes.

5. Return beef to skillet and add celery, tomatoes, garlic, sea salt and bay leaf.
6. Add pepper and 2 tablespoons water, cover and cook for 10 minutes.
7. Mix arrowroot with water.
8. Combine arrowroot mixture with other ingredients and cook for an additional 3 minutes.

Wild Rice

Health Benefits of Wild Rice: Wild rice is high in protein and fiber. A serving of wild rice gives more protein, B vitamins and zinc, and less starch than a similar serving of brown rice. Wild rice is used as a grain. However it is not really a grain. Wild rice is the seed of a water grass, and its nutty flavor enhances salads, soups, stir fries and side dishes.

Wild Rice Pilaf

<u>Serves 5</u>

1 lb wild rice
1 lb chicken, preferably free range
1 teaspoon oregano
2 sprigs thyme
4 cloves garlic, cleaned, washed and crushed
3 stalks celery, sliced and diced
3 carrots, cleaned, washed and diced
½ lb tomatoes, washed and diced
½ cup fresh or frozen green beans
1 medium onion
2 tablespoons unrefined coconut oil, unrefined olive oil or butter
¼ teaspoon black pepper
Salt to taste
3 pints
8 cups water

* * * *

1. Pour water in a pot and add salt to taste.
2. Bring to the boil, add rice and cook for about 30 minutes.
3. Clean and cut chicken in small pieces and marinate for about 1 hour with oregano, thyme, and garlic.

4. Lightly sauté onion in oil in a skillet, add chicken and cook for 10 minutes, stirring constantly.
5. Add celery, carrots, tomatoes, beans and pepper to chicken mixture.
6. Add vegetable/chicken mixture to cooked rice and mix in.
7. Cover and cook for an additional 10 minutes on low heat.

Strategic Steps to a Healthier You

1. Take a Daily Dosage of Vitamin D

- More than 6,000 IU if you are suffering from a chronic disease
- More than 5,000 IU if you are 65 years or older
- 6,000 IU if you are pregnant
- 5,000 IU for teens and adults of normal health
- 2,500 IU for children 5-12 years of age
- 35 units per pound for children 5 years and younger

Bear in mind that you may need more than the required daily amounts if you are dark-skinned and if you are obese. Also, remember that it is important to have your vitamin D levels checked every 6-12 months to ensure that you maintain optimal levels between 50 and 100 nanograms per milliliter (ng/ml).

2. Exercise

- Exercise at least 4 days per week.
- Fat burning exercise, especially muscle-building exercise, boosts your vitamin D levels.
- Make your exercise routine fun and you are more likely to stick with it.

3. Choose Whole Foods Instead of Processed Foods

- Eat ample servings of fresh, organic vegetables and fruits daily.
- Eat hormone-free, grass-fed meats.
- Eat dairy products from pastured animals. Visit the Cornucopia Institute's website for reports on factory farm,

mass produced dairy products that you should avoid. They also provide a list of authentic free-range dairies and dairy products.

Guide to Resources

The list of resources outlined below is given to you as a guide to help you find some useful information. This list is by no means complete because it is impossible to list all the reputable nutrition and health resources that are available to you. However, you may go to the website www.healthieryounutrition.com to find additional information on resources discussed in this book.

1. The *Vitamin D Council,* www.vitamindcouncil.org increases public and professional awareness of the health benefits of vitamin D.

2. The Sunlight, Nutrition, and Health Research Center, www.sunarc. org is devoted to research and education relating to prevention of chronic diseases through changes in diet and lifestyle. Special emphasis is placed on the beneficial role of UVB radiation in health.

3. www.pubmed.gov is a service of the US National Library of Medicine, comprising more than 20 million citations from biomed fields. Literature comes from MEDLINE, life science, journals and online books, and may include publisher websites.

4. www.healthresearchforum.org.uk develops and disseminates information in order to improve public health in the United Kingdom.

5. About 1,500 chemicals - pesticides are used to kill insects, fungi, worms, and rodents. Your foods may be exposed to these dangerous chemicals. Free Complete Shoppers Guides to pesticides are available at http://www.foodnews.org/wallet guide.php

6. For reputable producers of locally grown foods in your area go to www.localharvest.org

7. The website www.eatwild.com lists reputable providers of grass fed meats.

8. Visit www.seafoodwatch.org for detailed information on seafood recommendations.

9. To get information about factory farm mass-produced eggs versus authentic free range eggs go to http://www.cornucopia. org/2010/09/organic-egg-report-and-scorecard/

10. The non-gmo food shopping guide may be obtained for free at http://www. nongmoshoppingguide.com

11. An active lifestyle contributes to a healthy weight. You may find suggestions for exercise activities for children and adults at www.letsmove.gov

12. Juicers. Visit www.healthieryounutrition.com for juicer recommendations.

13. Water Filters. For good quality water filter recommendations, visit www.healthieryounutrition.com.

Selected Bibliography

Chapter One: Rays of Life

Benefits of Sunlight: A Bright Spot for Human Health. *Environmental Health Perspective* 2008;116(4):A162-A167.

Byremo G, Red G, Carlsen KH. Effect of Climatic Change in Children with Atopic Eczema. *Allergy* 2006;61:1403-1410.

Fox J, Peters B, Prakash M, Arribas J, Hill A, Moecklinghoff C. Improvement in Vitamin D Deficiency Following Antiretroviral Regime Change: Results from the MONET Trial. *Aids Research Human Retroviruses* 2010;PMID:20854196.

Gille O. A New Government Policy is Needed for Sunlight and Vitamin D. *British Journal of Dermatology* 2006;154(6):1052-1061.

Grant WB. In Defense of the Sun: An Estimate of Change in Mortality Rates in the United States if mean Serum 25-hydroxyvitamin D levels were raised to 45 ng/ml by Solar Ultraviolet-B Irradiance. *Dermato-Endocrinology* 2009;1(4):207-214.

Kong S, Lee D, Kwak S, Kim J, Sohn J, Kim I. Characterization of Sunlight-grown Transgenic Rice Plants Expressing Arabdopsis phytochrome A. *Molecular Breeding* 2004;14:35-45.

Lambert GW, Reid C, Kaye DM. et. al. Effect of Sunlight and Season on Serotonin Turnover in the Brain. *Lancet 2002;*360:9348.

Lampe F, Snyder S. Conversation with Michael Holick, PHD, MD: Vitamin D Pioneer. Alternative *Therapies* 2008;14(3):65-75.

Mitakakis TZ, O'meara TJ, Tovey ER. The Effect of Sunlight on Allergen Release from Spores of the Fungus Alternaria. *Grana* 2003;42:43-46.

Mehrdad, S. Prevalence of Vitamin D Deficiency among Female Students in Secondary Guidance School in Yazd City. *Acta Medica Iranica* 2009;47(3):209-214.

Plotnikoff G A, Quigley JM. Prevalence of Severe Hypovitaminosis D in Patients with Persistent, Nonspecific Musculoskeletal Pain. *Mayo Clinic Proceedings 2003;*78 (12):1463-1470.

Reinhardt K, Smith WK, Carter GA. Clouds and Cloud Immersion Alter Photosynthetic Light Quality in a Temperate Mountain Cloud Forest. *Botany* 2010;88:462-470.

Stokstad E. The Vitamin D Deficit. *Science* 2003;302(5652):6-10.

Swetha S, Santhosh SM, Balakrishna RG. Enhanced Bacterial Activity of Modified Titania in Sunlight against Pseudomonas aeruginosa, a water-borne Pathogen. *Photochemistry and Photobiology* 2010; 86:1127-1134.

Tangpricha V. Vitamin D Deficiency in the Southern United States. *Southern* Medical *Journal* 2007 April;100(4):384-385.

Unger MD, Cuppari L, Titan SM, Magalhaes MC, Sassaki AL, Dos Reis LM. Vitamin D Status in a Sunny Country: Where has the Sun Gone? *Clinical Nutrition 2010;PMID:20637530.*

Williams WE, Gordon HL, Witiak SM. Chloroplasts Movements in the Field. *Plant Cell and Environment* 2003;26:2005-2014.

Yamada M, Kawasaki M, Sugiyama T, Miyake H, Taniguchi M. Differential Positioning of C4 Mesophyll and Bundle sheath Chloroplasts: aggregative Movement of C4 Mesophyll Chloroplasts in Response to Environmental Stresses. *Plant Cell Physiology* 2009;50(10):1736-1749.

Chapter Two: Melanin and Vitamin D

Bhalla A. Vitamin D Deficiency. *General Practice Update* 2009;2(6):21-28.

Bibuld D. Health Disparities and Vitamin D. *Clinical Reviews in Bone and Mineral Metabolism* 2009 April;7:63-76.

Brom B. Vitamin Use in an Integrative Medical Practice: The New Roles of Vitamin D. *South African Family Practice* 2010 Jan-Feb;52(1):44-46.

Cannell JJ, Hollis BW. Use of Vitamin D in Clinical Practice. *Alternative Medicine Review* 2008;13(1):6-20.

Cronin SC. The Dual Vitamin D Pathways: Considerations for Adequate Supplementation. *Nephrology Nursing Journal* 2010;37(1):19-36.

Ferrie H. Nature's Magic Bullet. *The CCPM Monitor* 2009:12-15.

Garland CF, Gorham ED. Vitamin D for Cancer Prevention: Global Perspective. *Association of Educational Psychologists* 2009 July;19(7):468-83.

Gillie O. A New Government Policy is needed for Sunlight and Vitamin D. *British Journal of Dermatology* 2006;154(6):1052-1061.

Ginde AA, Liu MC, Camargo CA. Demographic Differences and Trends of Vitamin D Insufficiency in the US Population, 1988-2004. *Archive of Internal Medicine* 2009;169(6):626-632.

Grant WB. Differences in Vitamin-D Status may Explain Black-White Differences in Breast Cancer Survival Rates. *Journal of the National Medical Association* 2008 September;100(9):*1040.*

Grant WB, Holick MF. Benefits and Requirements of Vitamin D for Optimal Health: A Review. *Alternative Medicine Review* 2005; 10(2):94-105.

Grant WB, Mohr SB. Ecological Studies of Ultraviolet B, Vitamin D and Cancer Since 2000. *Association of Educational Psychologists* 2009;19(7):446-54.

Grant WB, Strange RC, Garland CF. Sunshine is Good Medicine. The Health Benefits of Ultra-violet-B Induced Vitamin D Production. *Journal of Cosmetic Dermatology* 2003;2(2):86-98.

Holick MF, Chen TC. Assessment of Vitamin D in Population-Based Studies – Vitamin D Deficiency: A Worldwide Problem with Health Consequences. *American Journal of Clinical Nutrition* 2008; 87(4):1080S-1086S.

Holick MF. High Prevalence of Vitamin D Inadequacy and Implications for Health. *Mayo Clinic Proceedings* 2006;81(3):353-373.

Jablonski NG, Chaplin G. Skin Deep. *Scientific American* 2002 October; 74-81.

Jablonski NG. 2008. *Skin: A Natural History*. Berkeley: University of California Press.

Lampe F, Snyder S. Conversation with Michael Holick, PHD, MD: Vitamin D Pioneer. Alternative *Therapies* 2008;14(3):65-75.

Millen AE, Bodnar LM. Vitamin D Assessment in Population-based Studies: A Review of the Issues. *American Journal of Clinical Nutrition* 2008;87(4):1102S-5S.

Chapter Three: Disproportionate Disease and Mortality Rates Among Blacks

Bennet B. Broadening Horizons: African American Consumers Seek Health, Adventure. *Stagnito's New Products Magazine* 2006.

Brand CA, Abi HY, Couch DE, Vindigni A, Wark JD. Vitamin D Deficiency: A Study of Community Beliefs among Dark-skinned and Veiled People. *International Journal of Rheumatic Diseases* 2008;11(1):15-23.

Brenner M, Hearing VJ. The Protective Role of Melanin Against UV Damage in Human Skin. *Photochemistry and Photobiology* 2008; 84:539-545.

Couzin J. Probing the Roots of Race and Cancer. *Science* 2007 Feb;315(5812):592-594.

Dong Y, Stallmann-Jorgensen IS, Pollock NK, Harris RA, Keeton D, Huang Y, Li K, Bassali R, *Guo D, Thomas J, Pierce GL, White J, Holick MF and Zhu H.* A 16-Week Randomized Clinical Trial of 2000 International Units Daily Vitamin D3 Supplementation in Black Youth: 25-Hydroxyvitamin D, Adiposity, and Arterial Stiffness. *The Journal of Clinical Endocrinology and Metabolism* 2010 July; 10:1210-1220.

Fiscella K, Franks P. Vitamin D, Race and Cardiovascular Mortality: Findings from a National U.S. Sample. *Annals of Family Medicine* 2010; 8:11-18.

Fiscella K, Franks P. Vitamin D, Race, and Cardiovascular Mortality: Vitamin D: A Bright Spot in Nutrition Research. *Harvard Heart Letter* 2010;3.

Ford LV, Graham A, Wall A, Berg J. Vitamin D Concentrations in an UK Inner-City Multicultural Outpatient Population. *Annals of Clinical Biochemistry* 2006;43:468-473.

Freedman BI, Wagenknecht LE, Hairston KG, Bowden DW, Carr JJ, Hightower RC, Gordon EJ, Xu J, Langefeld CD, Divers J. Vitamin D, Adiposity, and Calcified Atherosclerotic Plaque in African-Americans. *The Journal of Clinical Endocrinology and Metabolism* 2010;95(30):1076-1083.

Ginde AA, Liu MC, Camargo CA. Demographic Differences and Trends of Vitamin D Insufficiency in the U.S. Population, 1988-2004. *Archives of Internal Medicine* 2009;169:626-632.

Grant WB, Peiris AN. Possible Role of Serum 25-Hydroxyvitamin D in Black-White Health Disparities in the United States. *Journal of the American Medical Association* 2010 Nov;11(9):617-628.

Harris SS. Vitamin D and African Americans. *Journal of Nutrition* 2006;136(4):1126-1129.

Holick MF. 2010. *The Vitamin D Solution.* New York: Hudson Street Press.

Jablonski, NG, Chaplin G. Colloquium Paper: Human Skin Pigmentation as an Adaptation to UV Radiation. *Proceedings of the National Academy of Science* 2010;107(2):8962-8968.

Jablonski NG, Chaplin G. Skin Deep. *Scientific American* 2003;13(2).

Kyriakidou-Himonas M, Aloia JF, Yeh JK. Vitamin D Supplementation in Postmenopausal Black Women. *The Journal of Clinical Endocrinology & Metabolism* 1999;84(11):3988-90.

Lack of Vitamin D Causes Many Cancers And Diseases In African-Americans. *Oakland Post.* 2007 December 27-January;2,6.

Lack of Vitamin D Causes Many Cancers And Diseases In African-Americans But Vitamin D Pills Are An Available Remedy. *Oakland Post.* 2006 December 13;19,6.

McKinney K, Breitkopf CR, Berenson AB. Association of Race, Body Fat and Season with Vitamin D Status Among Young Women: A Cross-sectional Study. *Clinical Endocrinology* 2008 Oct;69(4):535-41.

Malatesta K, Norris K, Williams S. Vitamin D and Chronic Kidney Disease. *Ethnicity and Disease* 2009 Autumn;19(4):S5-8-S5-11.

Miyamura Y, Coelho SG, Wolber R, Miller SA, Wakamatsu K, Zmudzka BZ, Ito S, et. al. Regulation of Human Skin Pigmentation and Responses to Ultraviolet Radiation. *Pigment Cell Research* 2006;20:2-13.

Ortonne JP. Photo-protective Properties of Skin Melanin. *British Journal of Dermatology* 2002;146:7-10.

Rainville C, Khan Y, Tisman G. Triple Negative Breast Cancer Patients Presenting with Low Serum Vitamin D Levels: A Case Series. *Cases Journal* 2009;2:8390.

Rajakumar K, Fernstrom JD, Janosky JE, Greenspan SL. Vitamin D Insufficiency in Preadolescent African American Children. *Clinical Pediatrics* 2005;44:683-692.

Raloff J. Vitamin D: Blacks Need Much More. *Science News* 2007; 172(25/27).

Raloff J. Many Babies Born Short of Vitamin D. *Science News* 2007; 171(6).

Rostand SG. Vitamin D, Blood Pressure, and African Americans: Toward a Unifying Hypothesis. *Clinical Journal of American Society of Nephrology* 2010 Sept;5(9):1697-1703.

Scalzi LV, Bhatt S, Gilkeson RC, Schaffer ML. The Relationship Between Race, Cigarette Smoking and Carotid Intimal Medial Thickness in Systemic Lupus Erthematosus. *Lupus* 2009 Oct;18:1289-1297.

Schieszer J. Vitamin D Deficiency Linked to Low Bone Density in Black Men: Low Levels More Common than Previously Thought. *Internal Medicine World Report* 2007;11.

Schwartz GG. Vitamin D and the Epidemiology of Prostate Cancer. *Seminars in Dialysis* 2005;18(4):276-289.

Sewell, Douglas. Low Vitamin D Levels Put Blacks at Risk. *Michigan Chronicle* 2008 June 11-17;A5.

Stephensen J. African American Teens Seen Low in Vitamin D. *Agricultural Research* 2007; 41(2):23.

Stokstad, Erik. The Vitamin D Deficit. *Science* 2003Dec;302(5652):6-10.

Terrell AM. The Association of Vitamin D Receptor Polymorphism and the Risk of Diabetes in African American and Hispanic American Females. *Ethnicity and Disease* 2008;18(2):S1-88.

Trivers KF, Lund MJ, Porter PL, Lift JM, Flagg EW, Coates R J, Eley JW. *The* Epidemiology of Triple-Negative Breast Cancer,including Race. *Cancer Causes and Control 2009;20(7):1071-1082.*

Valina-Toth A, Lai Z, Quah R, Britton M, Yoo W, Flack JM. The Effects of Vitamin D and Parathyroid Hormone on Blood Pressure and Non-Invasively Measured Vascular Function in Normotensive African Americans. *Ethnicity and Disease* 2009 Autumn; 19(4):S4-4.

Wu SH, Ho SC, Zhong L. Effects of Vitamin D Supplementation on Blood Pressure. *Southern Medical Journal* 2010; 103(8):729-737.

Chapter Four: Vitamin D's Role in Preventing and Controlling Major Diseases: Immune Disorders

Adorini L, Penna G, Giarrantania N, Mariani R, Uskokovic MR. Inhibition of Type 1 Diabetes Development by D Receptor Antagonists. *Current Medicinal Chemistry* 2005;4(6):645-51.

Beretich B, Beretich T. Editorial regarding "Explaining Multiple Sclerosis Prevalence by Ultraviolet Exposure: a Geospatial Analysis". *Multiple Sclerosis* 2009;15:889-890.

Branisteanu DD. The Immune Modulating Effects of Vitamin D: How far are We from Clinical Applications? *Acta Endocrinologica (Buc)* 2006;2(4):437-55.

Brehm JM, Schuermann B, Fuhlbrigge AL, Hollis BW, Strunk RC, Zeiger RS, Weiss ST. Serum Vitamin D Levels and Severe Asthma Exacerbarions in the Childhood Asthma Management Program Study. *Journal Allergy & Clinical Immunology* 2010 July;126(1):52-58.

Cannell J, Hollis BW, Sorenson MB, Taft TN, Anderson JJB. Athletic Performance and Vitamin D. *Medicine and Science in Sports and Exercise.* 2009 May;41(5):102-10.

Cantorna MT. Vitamin D and Multiple Sclerosis: An Update. *Nutrition Reviews* 2008;66(2): S135-S138.

Chiuve SE, Korngold EC, Januzzi JL, Gantzer ML, Albert CM. Plasma and Dietary Magnesium and Risk of Sudden Cardiac Death in Women. *The American Journal of Clinical Nutrition* 2010 Nov;doi:10.3945.

Conesa-Botella A. Is Vitamin D Deficiency Involved in the Immune Reconstitution Inflammatory Syndrome? *AIDS Research and Therapy* 2009;6(4):1186-1190.

Evatt ML, DeLong MR, Kumari M, Auinger P, McDermott MP, Tangpricha V. High Prevalence Hypovitaminosis D Status in Patients with Early Parkinson Disease. *Archive of Neurology* 2011;68(3):314-319.

von Essen MR, Kongsbak M, Schjerling P, Olgaard K, Odum N, Geisler C. Vitamin D Controls T Cell Antigen Receptor Signaling and Activation of Human T Cells. *Nature Immunology* 2010;11:344-349.

Freishtat RJ, Igbal SF, Pillai DK, Klein CJ, Ryan LM, Benton AS, Teach SJ. High Prevalence of Vitamin D Deficiency among Inner-City African American Youth with Asthma in Washington, DC. *The Journal of Pediatrics* 2010;156(6):948-952.

Fox J, Peters B, Prakash M, Arribas J, Hill A, Moecklinghoff C. Improvement in Vitamin D deficiency Following Antiretroviral Regime Change: Results from the MONET Trial. *Aids Research Human Retroviruses* 2010;PMID:20854196.

Griffin, MD, Xing N, Kumar R. Vitamin D and Its Analogs as Regulators of Immune Activation and Antigen Presentation. *Annual Review of Nutrition* 2003;23:117-45.

Haagsman HP, Hogenkamp A, Eijk MV. Collectin-Mediated Innate Immune Defense in the Lung. *Journal of Organ Dysfunction* 2006;2:230-36.

Haber P. [Magnesium as a Food Supplement]. *Acta Med Austriaca* 2004 May;31(2):37-9.

Jatupol K, Freeman VL, Gerber BS, Geraci S. Association of A1C Levels with Vitamin D Status in U.S. Adults: Data from the National Health and Nutrition Examination Survey. *Diabetes Care* 2010 June; 33(6):1236-1238.

Jelinek, George A. Managing Multiple Sclerosis in Primary Care: Are we forgetting something? *Quality in Primary Care* 2009;17:55-61.

Keen C, Commisso J, Killip D, Ou C, Rognerud CL, Dennis K, Dunn JK. The Effect of a Marathon Run on Plasma and Urine Mineral and Metal Concentrations. *Journal of the American College of Nutrition* 1998 April;17(2):124-127.

Kuitert LM, Kletchko SL. Intravenous Magnesium sulphate in acute , life-threatening Asthma. *Annal of Emergency Medicine* 1991 Nov; 20(11):1243-1245.

Litonjua AA. Vitamin D and Asthma. *Respiratory Medicine* 2010;24(1):1-9.

May E, Khusru A, Zugel U. Immunoregulation through 1,25-Dihydroxyvitamin D3 and its Analogs. *Inflammation and Allergy* 2004;3:377-393.

Mehta S, Hunter D, Mugusi FM, Spiegelman D, Manji KP, Giovannucci EL, Hertzmark E, Msamanga GI, Fawzi WW. Perinatal Outcomes, Including Mother to Child Transmission of HIV, and Child Mortality and Their Association with Maternal Vitamin D Status in May Tanzania. *Journal of Infectious Diseases* 2009;200:1022-1030.

Mehta S, Hunter D, Mugusi FM, Spiegelman D, Manji KP, Giovannucci EL, Hertzmark E, Msamanga GI, Fawzi WW. Vitamin D Status of HIV-Infected Women and its Association with HIV Disease Progression, Anemia, and Mortality. *PLoS ONE* 2010 Jan;5(1):e8770:doi:101371.

Niino M, Fukazawa T, Toshiyuki S, Sasaki H. Therapeutic Potential of Vitamin D for Multiple Sclerosis. *Current Medicinal Chemistry* 2008;15:499-505.

Nouri-Aria KT, Durham SR. Regulatory T Cells and Allergic Disease. *Inflammation and Allergy* 2008;7:237-52.

Panajatovic M. Protective Role of Vitamin D as a Cellular Immuno-Modulator in Mycobacterium Tuberculosis-infected Health Care Workers. *South African Family Practice* 2009 Sept-Oct;51(1):434.

Parsons JP, Kaeding C, Phillips G, Jarjoura D, Wadley G, Mastronarde JG. Prevalence of Exercise-induced Bronchospasm in a Cohort of Varsity College Athlete. *Medicine and Science in Sports and Exercise* 2007;39(9):1487-1492.

Pugliatti M, Harbo HF, Holmøy T, Kampman MT, Myhr K-M, Riise T, Wolfson C. Haagsman Environmental Risk Factors in Multiple Sclerosis. *Acta Neurologica Scandinavica* 2009;117 (188):34-40.

Rouatbi S, Guandia F, Laatiri I, Tabka Z, Guenard H. Inhaled Fluoride, Magnesium Salt and L-arginine Reverse Bronchospasma. *Drug Testing Analysis* 2010 Feb;2(2):51-4.

Scalzi LV, Bhatt S, Gilkeson RC, Schaffer ML. The Relationship between Race, Cigarette Smoking and Carotid Intimal Medial Thickness in Systemic Lupus Erthematosus. *Lupus* 2009 Oct;18:1289-1297.

Sharan C, Halder SK, Thota C, Jaleel T, Nair S, Al-Hendy A. Vitamin D Inhibits Proliferation of Human Uterine Leiomyoma Cells via

Catechol-O-methyltransferase. *Fertility and Sterility* 2011 Jan;95(1): 247-253.

Strong C. Is Vitamin D a Ray of Hope for Patients with MS? *Neurology Reviews* 2009;17 (7):1.

Szodoray P, Nakken B, Gaal J, Jonsson R, Szegedi A, Zold E, Szegedi G, Brun JG, Gesztelyi R, Zeher M, Bodolay E. The Complex Role of Vitamin D in Autoimmune Diseases. *Scandinavian Journal of Immunology* 2008;68:261-269.

Wintergerst ES, Silvia M, Hornig DH. Contribution of Selected Vitamins and Trace Elements to Immune Function. *Annals of Nutrition and Metabolism* 2007;51:301-23.

Zhang D, Al-Hendy M, Richard-Davis G, Montgomery-Rice V, Sharan C, Rajaratnam V, Khurana A, Al-Hendy A. Green Tea Extract Inhibits Proliferation of Uterine Leiomyoma Cells in Vitro and in Nude Mice. *American Journal of Obstetrics and Gynecology* 2010 March; 202(3):289.el-289.e9.

Chapter Five: Vitamin D and Its Cofactors Help Prevent Heart Disease, Diabetes and Obesity

Almirall J, Vaquero M, Bare ML, Anton E. Association of Low Serum 25-Hydroxyvitamin D levels and High Arterial Blood Pressure in the Elderly. *Nephrology Dialysis Transplantation* 2009;25(2):503-509.

Beer TM, Venner PM, Ryan CW, Petrylak DP, Chatta G, Ruether JD, Chi KN, Curd JG, DeLougherty TG. High Dose Calcitriol May Reduce Thrombosis in Cancer Patients. *The British Journal of Haematology* 2006;135:392-394.

Bibbins-Domingo K, Pletcher MJ, Lin F, Vittinghoff E, Gardin JM, Arynchyn A, Lewis CE, Williams OD, Hulley SB. Racial Differences in Incident Heart Failure among Young Adults. *New England Journal of Medicine* 2009;360(12):1179-1190.

Bid HK, Konwar R, Aggarwal CG, Gautam S, Saxena, M, Nayak VL, Banerjee M. Vitamin D Receptor (FOKI, BSMI and TAQI) Gene Polymorphisms and Type 2 Diabetes Mellitus: A North Indian Study. *Indian Journal of Medical Sciences* 2009;63(5):187-194.

Chacko SA, Song Y, Nathan L, Tinker L, de Boer IH, Tylavsky F, Wallace R, Liu S. Relations of Dietary Magnesium Intake to Biomarkers of Inflammation and Endothelial Dysfunction in an Ethnically Diverse Cohort of Postmenopausal Women. *Diabetes Care* 2010 Feb; 33(2):304-310.

Dobnig H, Pilz S, Scharnagl H, Renner W, Seelhorst U, Wellnitz B, Kinkeldei J, Boehmn BO, Weihrauch G, Maerz W. Independent Association of Low Serum 25-Hydroxyvitamin D and 1,25-Dihydroxy vitamin D Levels with All-Cause and Cardiovascular Mortality. *Archives of Internal Medicine* 2008 June;168(12):340-1349.

Finklea JD, Grossman RE, Tangpricha V. Vitamin D and Chronic Lung Disease: A Review of Clinical Mechanisms and Clinical Studies. *Advances in Nutrition* 2011 May;2:244-253.

Fiscella K, Franks P. Vitamin D, Race and Cardiovascular Mortality: Findings from a National U.S. Sample. *Annals of Family Medicine* 2010;8:11-18.

Fiscella K, Franks P. Vitamin D, Race, and Cardiovascular Mortality: Vitamin D: A Bright Spot in Nutrition Research. *Harvard Heart Letter* 2010;3.

Freedman BI, Wagenknecht LE, Hairston KG, Bowden DW, Carr JJ, Hightower RC, Gordon EJ, Xu J, Langefeld CD, Divers J. Vitamin D, Adiposity, and Calcified Atherosclerotic Plaque in African-Americans. *The Journal of Clinical Endocrinology and Metabolism* 2010;95(30):1076-1083.

Kilkkinen A, Knekt P, Aro A, Rissanen H, Marniemi J, Heliövaara M. Vitamin D Status and the Risk of Cardiovascular Disease Death. *American Journal of Epidemiology* 2009;170(8): 1032-1039.

Krueger T, Westenfeld R, Schurgers L, Brandenburg V. Coagulation meets Calcification: the Vitamin K System. *International Journal of Artificial Organs* 2009 February;32(2):67-74.

Ligia AM and Wood RJ. Vitamin D and Blood Pressure Connection: Update on Epidemiological, Clinical, and Mechanistic Evidence. *Nutrition Reviews* 2008;66(5):291-297.

LindQvist PG, Epstein E, Olsson H. Does an Active Sun Exposure Habit Lower the Risk of Venous Thrombotic Events? A D-lightful Hypothesis. *Journal of Thrombosis and Haemostasis* 2009;7:605-610.

Lott AM. Managing Diabetes. *Black Enterprise* 2009;40(4).

McKinney K, Breitkopf CR, Berenson AB. Association of Race, Body Fat and Season with Vitamin D Status Among Young Women: A Cross-sectional Study. *Clinical Endocrinology* 2008 Oct;69(4):535-41.

Malatesta K, Norris K, Williams S. Vitamin D and Chronic Kidney Disease. *Ethnicity and Disease* 2009 Autumn;19(4):S5-8-S5-11.

Martini LA, Wood RJ. Vitamin D and Blood Pressure Connection: Update on Epidemiological, Clinical and Mechanistic Evidence. *Nutrition Reviews 2008;66(5):291–297.*

May HT, Bair TL, Lappe DL, Anderson JL, Horne BD, Calquist JF, Muhlestein JB. Association of Vitamin D Levels with Incident Depression among a General Cardiovascular Population. *American Heart Journal* 2010;159(6):1037-1043.

Mheid IA, Patel R, Murrow J, Morris A, Aznaouridis K, Rahman A, Fike L, Kadtaradze N, Ahmed Y, Uphoff I, Hooper C, Tangpricha V, Alexander RW, Brigham K, Quyyumi A. Vitamin D Status is Associated with Arterial Stiffness and Vascular Dysfunction in Healthy Humans. *Journal of the American College of Cardiology* 2011;57:2049,doi:10.1016/S0735-1097(11)62049-4.

Miller J, Rosenbloom A, Silverstein J. Childhood Obesity. *The Journal of Clinical Endocrinology and Metabolism* 2004;89(9):4211-4218.

Palomer X, Gonzalez-Clemente JM, Blanco-Vaca F, Mauricio D. Role of Vitamin D in the Pathogenesis of type 2 Diabetes Mellitus. *Diabetes, Obesity and Metabolism* 2008;10:185-197.

Pittas AG, Chung M, Trikalinos T, Mitri J, Brendel M, et.al. Systematic Review: Vitamin D and Cardiometabolic Outcomes. *Annals of Internal Medicine* 2010;52(5):307-320.

Rodriguez-Rodriguez E, Navia B, Lopez-Sobaler AM. Ortega RM. Vitamin D in Overweight/Obese Women and Its Relationship with Dietetic and Anthropometric Variables. *Obesity* 2009;17(4):778-782.

Rogers SA. M.D. 2005. *The High Blood Pressure Hoax.* Sarasota, FL: Sand Key Company, Inc.

Seyoum B, Seraj ES, Saenz C, Abdulkadir J. Hypomagnesemia in Ethiopians with Diabetes Mellitus. *Ethnicity and Disease* 2008 spring;18:147-151.

Siddiqui SMK, Chang E, Li J, Burglage C, Zou M, Buhman-S KK, Koser S, Donkin SS, Teegarden D. Dietary Intervention with Vitamin D, Calcium, and Whey Protein Reduced Fat Mass and Increased Lean Mass in Rats. *Nutrition Research* 2008 November;28(11):783-790.

Sun X , Zemel MB. 1, 25-Dihydroxyvitamin D and Corticosteroid Regulate Adipocyte Nuclear Vitamin D Receptor. *International Journal of Obesity* 2008;32:1305-1311.

Tarcin O, Yavuz DG, Ozben B, Telli A. Effect of Vitamin D Deficiency and Replacement on Endothelial Function in Asymptomatic Subjects. *The Journal of Clinical Endocrinology and Metabolism* 2009; 94(10):4023-4030.

Terrell AM. The Association of Vitamin D Receptor Polymorphism and the Risk of Diabetes in African American and Hispanic American Females. *Ethnicity and Disease* 2008;18(2):S1-88.

Valina-Toth ALB, Lai Z, Quah R, Britton M, Yoo W, Flack JM. The Effects of Vitamin D and Parathyroid Hormone on Blood Pressure and Non-Invasively Measured Vascular Function in Normotensive African Americans. *Ethnicity and Disease* 2009 Autumn;19(4):S4-4.

Valina-Toth ALB, Lai Z, Yoo W, Abou-Samra A, Gadegbeku CA, Flack JM. Relationship of Vitamin D and Parathyroid Hormone with Obesity and Body Composition in African Americans. *Clinical Endocrinology* 2010;72(5):595-603.

Von Hurst PR, Stonehouse W, Coad J. Insulin Sensitivity is improved with Vitamin D Supplementation in South Asian Women who are Vitamin D Deficient and Insulin Resistant – a randomized, placebo-controlled trial. *Australian Medical Journal* 2010 Feb;2(1):55-56.

Wallin R, Wajih N, Greenwood GT, Sane DC. Arterial Calcification: A Review of Mechanisms, Animal Models, and the Prospects for Therapy. *Medical Research Review* 2001 July;21(4):274-301.

Wang L, Manson JE, Song Y, Sesso HD. Systemic Review: Vitamin D and Calcium Supplementation in Prevention of Cardiovascular Events. *Annals of Internal Medicine* 2010;15:2428.

Wu SH, Ho SC, Zhong L. Effects of Vitamin D Supplementation on Blood Pressure. *Southern Medical Journal* 2010;103(8):729-737.

Chapter Six: Vitamin D Prevents Cancer Development and Growth

Allen IT, Gillett DS, Hamed H, Fentiman IS. Prognosis of Synchronous Bilateral Breast Cancer. *British Journal of Surgery* 2009;96:376-380.

Alvarez-Diaz S, Valle N, Garcia JM. Cystatin D is a Candidate Tumor Suppressor Gene Induced by Vitamin D in Human Colon Cancer Cells. *The Journal of Clinical Investigation* 2009;119(8):2343-58.

Beer TM, Venner PM, Ryan CW, Petrylak DP, Chatta G, Ruether JD, Chi KN, Curd JG, DeLougherty TG. High Dose Calcitriol May Reduce Thrombosis in Cancer Patients. *The British Journal of Haematology* 2006;135:392-394.

Bertone-Johnson ER. Vitamin D and Breast Cancer. *Association of Educational Psychologists* 2009;19(7):462-67.

Crew KD, Shane E, Creners S, McMahon DJ, Irani D, Hershman DL. High Prevalence of Vitamin D Deficiency Despite Supplementation in Premenopausal Women with Breast Cancer Undergoing Adjuvant

Chemotherapy. *American Journal of Oncology* 2009 May;27(3): 2151-2156.

Davies EA, Linklater KM, Coupland VH, Toy J, Park R, Petit J, Housden C, Moller H. *British* Investigation of 5-Year relative Survival for Breast Cancer in a London Cancer Network. *Journal of Cancer* 2010 Sept;103:1076-1080.

Davies L, Welch HG. Increasing Incidence of Thyroid Cancer in the United States, 1973-2002. *Journal of the American Medical Association* 2006;295:2164-2167.

Eliassen AH, Spiegelman D, Hollis BW, Horst RL, Willett WC, Hankinson SE. Plasma 25-hydroxyvitamin D and Risk of Breast Cancer in the Nurses' Health Study II. *Breast Cancer Res*earch 2011 May 11;13(3): R50. [Epub ahead of print]

Fakih MG, Trump DL, Johnson CS, Tian L, Muindi J, Sunga AY. Chemotherapy is Linked to Severe Vitamin D Deficiency in Patients with Colorectal Cancer. *International Journal of Colorectal Diseases* 2009;24:219-224.

Fang F, Kasperzyk JL, Shui I, Hendrickson W, Hollis BW, Fall K, Ma J, Gaziano JM, Stampfer MJ, Mucci LA, Giovannucci E. Prediagnostic Plasma Vitamin D Metabolites and Mortality among Patients with Prostate Cancer. *PloS One* 2011 April;6(4):e18625.

Fuzikawa AK, Peixoto SV, Taufer M, Moriguchi EH, Lima-Costa MF. Apolipoprotein E Study: Polymorphism Distribution in an Elderly Brazillian Population in the Bambui Health and Aging Study. *Brazillian Journal of Medical and Biological Research* 2007 Nov; 40(11):1429-1434.

Garland CF, French CB, Baggerly LL, Heaney RP. Vitamin D Supplement Doses and Serum 25- Hydroxyvitamin D in the Range Associated with Cancer Prevention. *Anticancer Research* 2011;31:617-622.

Garland CF, Gorham ED, Mohr SB, Garland FC. Vitamin D for Cancer Prevention: Global Perspective. *Annals of Epidemiology* 2009 April; 1047-2797.

Grant WB. Weighing the evidence linking UVB Irradiance, vitamin D, and Cancer Risk. *Mayo Clinic Proceedings* 2011 Apr;86(4):362-363.

Grant WB. Additional strong evidence that optimal serum 25(OH)D levels are at least 75 nmol/l. *International Journal of Epidemiology* 2011 April Epub; doi: 10.1093/ije/dyr068

Grant WB. The Roles of Ultraviolet-B Irradiance, Vitamin D, Apolipoprotein E ε4 and Diet in the Risk of Prostate Cancer. *Cancer Causes Control* 2010 Oct;22:157-158.

Grant WB. A Multicountry Ecological Study of Risk-modifying Factors for Prostate Cancer: Apolipoprotein E ε4 as a Risk Factor and Cereals as a Risk Reduction Factor. *Anticancer Research* 2010 Jan;30(1):189-199.

Grant WB. Official Recommended Intake for Vitamin D is Too Low: 2,000 IU/Day or More Needed for Optimal Health. *Orthomolecular Medicine News Service* 2010 February 19.

Grant WB. How Strong is the Evidence that Solar Ultraviolet B and Vitamin D Reduce the Risk of Cancer? An Examination using Hill's Criteria for Casuality. *Dermato-Endocrinology* 2009:1(1):17-24.

Grant WB. Differences in Vitamin-D Status may Explain Black-White Differences in Breast Cancer Survival Rates. *Journal of the National Medical Association* 2008 September;100(9):*1040.*

Grant WB. Lower Vitamin-D Production from Solar Ultraviolet-B Irradiance May Explain Some Differences in Cancer Survival Rates. *Journal of the National Medical Association* 2006 March;98(3):357-364.

Haiman CA, Stram DO, Wilkens LR, Pike MC, Kolonel LN, Henderson BE, Marchand L. Ethnic and Racial Differences in the Smoking-Related Risk of Lung Cancer. *N Engl J Medicine* 2006 Jan;354(4):333-42.

Hines SL, Jorn HK, Thompson KM, Larson JM. Breast Cancer Survivors and Vitamin D: A Review. *Nutrition* 2010 March;26(3):255-262.

Irvine T, Allen DS, Gillett H, Hamed I, Fentiman S. Prognosis of Synchronous Bilateral Breast Cancer. *British Journal of Surgery* 2009;96:376-380.

Jenab M, Bueno-de-Mesquita H, Ferrari P, van Duijnhoven FJB, Norat T, Pischon T, Jansen EHJM, Slimani N, Byrnes G, Rinaldi S, Tjonneland A, Olsen A, Overvad K, Boutron- Ruault M, Clavel-Chapelon F, Morois S, Kaaks R, Linseisen J, Boeing H, Bergmann MM, Trichopoulou A, Misirli G, Trichopoulou D, Berrino F, Vineis P, Panico S, Palli D, Tumino R, Ros MM, van Gils CH, Peeters PH, Brustad M, Tormo M, Ardanaz E, Rodriguez L, Sanchez M, Dorronsoro M, Gonzalez CA, Hallsmans G, Palmqvist R, Roddam A, Key TJ, Khaw K, Autier P, Hainaut P, Riboli E. Association Between pre-Diagnostic Circulating Vitamin D Concentration and Risk of Colorectal Cancer in European populations: A nested Case control study. *British Medical Journal* 2010;340:b5500.

Kaiser U, Schilli M, Wegmann B, Barth P, Wedel S, Hofmann J, Havemann K. Expresssion of Vitamin D Receptor in Lung Cancer. *J Cancer Resp Clin Oncology* 1996;122: 356-359.

Khalsa S. 2009. *The Vitamin D Revolution.* Carlsbad, California: Hay House, Inc.

Khan QJ, Fabian CJ. How I Treat Vitamin D Deficiency. *Journal of Oncology Practice* 2010;6(2):97-101.

Lack of Vitamin D Causes Many Cancers and Diseases In African-Americans. *Oakland Post.* 2007 December 27- January; 2,6.

Lappe JM, Travers-Gustafson D, Davies KM, Recker RR, Heaney RP Vitamin D and Calcium Supplementation reduces Cancer Risk: Results of a Randomized Trial. *American Journal of Clinical Nutrition* 2007;85(6):1586-1591.

Lee JE, Li H, Chan AT, Hollis BW, Lee IM, Stampfer MJ, Wu K, Giovannucci E, Ma J. Circulating Levels of Vitamin D and Colon and Rectal Cancer: The Physicians' Health Study and a Meta-analysis of Prospective Studies. *Cancer Prevention Research* (Phila) 2011 May;4(5):735-43.

Lim HS, Roychoudhuri R, Peto J, Schwartz G, Baade P, Moller H. Cancer Survival is Dependent on Season of Diagnosis and Sunlight Exposure. *International Journal of Cancer* 2006;119(7):1530-1536.

Mohr SB, Garland CF, Gorham ED, Grant WB, Garland FC. Relationship Between Low Ultraviolet B Irradiance and Higher Breast Cancer Risk in 107 Countries. *The Breast Journal* 2008;14(3):255-260.

Ng K, Sargent DJ, Goldberg RM, Meyerhardt JA, Green EM, Pitot HC, Hollis BW, Pollak MN, Fuchs CS. Vitamin D Status in Patients with Stage IV Colorectal Cancer: Findings from Intergroup Trial N9741. *Journal of Clinical Oncology* 2011 April;29(12):1599-1606.

Ng K, Wolpin BM, Meyerhardt JA, Wu K, Chan AT, Hollis BW, Giovannucci EL, Stampfer MJ. Prospective Study of Predictors of Vitamin D Status and Survival in Patients with Colorectal Cancer. *British Journal of Cancer* 2009;101:916-923.

Rainville C, Khan Y, Tisman G. Triple Negative Breast Cancer Patients Presenting with Low Serum Vitamin D Levels: A Case Series. *Cases Journal* 2009.

Schwartz GG. Vitamin D and the Epidemiology of Prostate Cancer. *Seminars in Dialysis* 2005;18 (4):276-289.

Society of Integrative Oncology, quoting Kathy Crew, Gregory A. Plotnikoff and Michael Holick http://www.integrativeonc.org/index. php/institute-of-medicine-report-on-vitamin-d

Spreen A. *Vitamin D Conspiracy leads straight to Big Pharma.* 02/19/2011 http://www.healthiertalk.com/vitamin-d-conspiracy-leads-straight-big-pharma-3396

Stead LA, Lash TL, Sobieraj JE, Chi DD, Westrup JL, Charlot M, Blanchard RA, Lee JC, King TC, Rosenberg CL. Triple-Negative Breast Cancers Are Increasing in Black Women Regardless of Age or Body Index. *Breast Cancer Research* 2009;**11**:R18doi:10.1186/bcr2242http: breast-cancer-research.com/content/11/2/R18.

Tangpricha V, Spina C, Yao M, Chen TC, Wolfe MM, Holick M. Vitamin D Deficiency Enhances the Growth of MC-26 Colon Cancer Xenografts in Balb/c Mice. *The Journal of Nutrition* 2005;135:2350-2354.

Thun MJ, Hannan LM, Adams-Campbell LL, Boffetta P, Buring JE, et al. Lung Cancer Occurrence in Never-Smokers: An Analysis of 13 Cohorts and 22 Cancer Registry Studies. *PloS Medicine* 2008 Sept; 5(8):e185.

Too Many Cases, Too Many Deaths: Lung Cancer in African Americans. *American Lung Association Disparities in Lung Health Series* 2010:1-22.

Trivers KF, Lund MJ, Porter PL, Lift JM, Flagg EW, Coates RJ, Eley JW. The Epidemiology of Triple-Negative Breast Cancer, including Race. *Cancer Causes and Control 2009;20(7):1071-1082.*

Wei Z, Suk R, Liu G, Park S, Neuberg DS, Wain JC, Lynch TJ, Giovannucci E, Christiani DC. Vitamin D is associated with Improved Survival in early-stage Non-small cell Lung Cancer Patients. *Cancer Epidemiol Biomarkers Prev* 2005 Oct;14(10):2303-9.

Win T, Sharples L, Groves AM, Ritchie AJ, Wells FC, Laroche CM. Predicting Survival in Potentially Curable Lung Cancer Patients. *Lung* 2008;186:97-102.

Zhou W, Heist RS, liu G, Neuberg DS, Asomaning K, Su L, Wain JC, Lynch TJ, Giovannucci E, Christiani DC. Polymorphisms of Vitamin D Receptor and Survival in Early Stage Non-small Cell Lung Cancer Patients. *Cancer Epidemiology Prevention* 2006 Nov;15(11)2239-45.

Zinser GM, Welsh JE. Vitamin D Receptor Status Alters Mammary Gland Morphology and Tumorigenesis in MMTV- neu mice. *Carcinogenesis* 2004;25:2361-2372.

Chapter Seven: Mood Disorders

Dealberto MJ. Ethnic Origin and Increased Risk for Schizophrenia in Immigrants to Countries of Recent and Longstanding Immigration. *Acta Psychiatrica Scandinavica* 2010;121(5):325-339.

Eyles DW, Smith S, Kinobe R, Hewinson M, McGrath JJ. Distribution of the Vitamin D Receptor And 1-alpha-hydroylase in Human Brain. *Journal of Chemical Neuroanatomy* 2005;29:21-30.

Eyles D, Cui X, Pelekanos M, Kesby J, Burne T, Mcgrath J. S67-03 Developmental Vitamin D Deficiency (DVD) and Brain Dopamine Ontogeny. *European Psychiatry* 2009;24(1):S319- S330.

Garcion E, Wion-Barbot N, Montero-Menei CN, Berger F, Wion D. New Clues about Vitamin D Functions in the Nervous System. *Trends Endocrinology and Metabolism* 2002 Apr;13(3):100-105.

Hoogendijk WJG, Lips P, Dik MG, Deej DJH, Beekman ATF, Penninx BWJH. Depression is Associated With Decreased 25-Hydroxyvitamin D and Increased Parathyroid Hormone Levels in Older Adults. *Archives of General Psychiatry* 2008;65(5):508-512.

Humble MB. Vitamin D, Light and Mental Health. *Journal of Photochemistry and Photobiology* 2010 November 3;101(2):142-149.

Jorde R, Sneve M, Figenschau Y, Svartberg J, Waterloo K. Effects of Vitamin D Supplementation on Symptoms of Depression in Overweight and Obese Subjects: Randomized Double Blind Trial. *Journal of Internal Medicine* 2008;264(6):599-609.

Kesby JP, Cui X, Ko P, McGrath JJ, Burne THJ, Eyles DW. Developmental Vitamin D Deficiency Alters Dopamine Turnover in Neonatal Rat Forebrain. *Neuroscience Letters 2009;*461(2):155-158.

Lambert GW, Reid C, Kaye DM, Jennings GL, Esler MD. Effect of Sunlight and Season on Serotonin Turnover in the Brain. *Lancet* 2002 Dec; 360(9348):1840-1842.

McCann J, Ames B. Is there Convincing Biological or *Behavioral* Evidence Linking Vitamin D Deficiency to Brain Dysfunction? *The FASEB Journal* 2008;22(4):982-1001.

McGrath JJ, Eyles DW, Pendersen CB. Neonatal Vitamin D Status and Risk of Schizophrenia. *Archive of General Psychiatry* 2010;67(9): 889-894.

McGrath JJ, Eyles DW, Mowry B, Yolken R, Buka S. Low Maternal Vitamin D as a Risk Factor for Schizophrenia: A Pilot Study Using Banked Sera. *Schizophrenia Research* 2003;63:73-78

May HT, Bair TL, Lappe DL, Anderson JL, Horne BD, Calquist JF, Muhlestein JB. Association of Vitamin D Levels with Incident Depression among a General Cardiovascular Population. *American Heart Journal* 2010;159(6):1037-1043.

Milaneshi Y, Shardell M, Corsi AM, Vazzana R, Bandinelli S, Guralnik JM, Ferrucci L. Serum 25-Hydroxyvitamin D and Depressive Symptoms in Older Women and Men. The Journal of Clinical Endocrinology and Metabolism 2010;95(7):3225-3233.

Murphy PK, Wagner CL. Vitamin D and Mood Disorders among women: An Integrative Review. *Journal Midwifery Women's Health* 2008 Sept;53(5):440-446.

Plotnikoff G A, Quigley JM. Prevalence of Severe Hypovitaminosis D in Patients with Persistent, Nonspecific Musculoskeletal Pain. *Mayo clinic Proceedings* 2003;78 (12):1463-1470.

Wilkins CH, Birge SJ, Sheline YI, Morris JC. Vitamin D Deficiency Affects Worse Cognitive Performance and Lower Bone Density in Older African Americans. *Journal of National Medical Association* 2009 April;101(4):349-54.

Chapter Eight: Special Vitamin D Needs of Elderly Blacks and Institutionalized Blacks

Almirall J, Vaquero M, Bare ML, Anton E. Association of Low Serum 25-Hydroxyvitamin D levels and High arterial Blood Pressure in the Elderly. *Nephrology Dialysis Transplantation* 2009;25(2):503-509.

Barake R. Vitamin D supplement Consumption is Required to Achieve Minimal Target 25- Hydroxyvitamin D Concentration of greater than 75 nmol/L in older people. *Journal of Nutrition* 2010;140(3): 551-556.

Cardinal RN, Gregory CA. Osteomalacia and Vitamin D Deficiency in a Psychiatric Rehabilitation Unit: Case Report and Survey. *BioMed Research* 2009;2(82):50-57.

Chatfield SM, Brand C, Ebling PR, Russell DM. Vitamin D Deficiency in General Medical Inpatients in Summer and Winter. *Internal Medical Journal* 2007;37(6):377-382.

Cheng S, Massaro JM, Fox CS, Larson MG, Keyes MJ, McCabe EL, Robins SJ, et. al. Adiposity, Cardiometabolic Risk, and Vitamin D Status: The Framingham Heart Study. *Diabetes* 2010;59(1):242-249.

Cherniack EP, Levis S, Troen BR. Hypovitaminosis D: A Stealthy Epidemic that Requires Treatment. *Geriatrics* 2008;63(4):24-30.

Djoussé L, Arnett DK, Coon H, Province MA, Moore LL, Ellison RC. Fruit and vegetable consumption and LDL cholesterol: the National Heart, Lung, and Blood Institute Family Heart Study. *American Journal of Clinical Nutrition* 2004 Feb;79(2):213-217.

Formiga F, Ferrer A, Riera-Mestre A, Chivite D, Nolla JM, Pujol R. High Percentage of Vitamin D Deficiency in Nonagenarians. *Journal of American Geriatrics Society* 2008;56(11):2147-2148.

Fritz K, Ibrahim E. Quality of Nutrition of Elderly with Different Degrees of Dependency: Elderly Living in Private Homes. *Annals of Nutrition and Metabolism* 2008;52(1):47-50.

Ginde AA, Camargo CA, Shapiro NI. Vitamin D Insufficiency and Sepsis Severity in Emergency Department Patients with Suspected Infection. *Academic Emergency Medicine* 2011;18:1-4.

Grant WB. Official Recommended Intake for Vitamin D is Too Low: 2,000 IU/Day or More Needed for Optimal Health. *Orthomolecular Medicine News Service* 2010 February 19.

Grant WB. Does Vitamin D Reduce the Risk of Dementia? *Journal of Alzheimer's Disease* 2009;17:151-159.

Hirani V, Ali A, Mindell J. Urgent Action Needed to Improve Vitamin D Status Among Older People in England. *Age and Ageing* 2010;39(1): 62-68.

Jatupol K, Freeman VL, Gerber BS, Geraci S. Association of A1C Levels with Vitamin D Status in U.S. Adults: Data from the National Health and Nutrition Examination Survey. *Diabetes Care* 2010 June;33(6): 1236-1238.

Jeng L, Yamshchikov AV, Judd SE, Blumberg HM, Martin GS, Ziegler TR, Tangpricha V. Alterations in Vitamin D Status and Anti-microbial Peptide Levels in Patients in the Intensive Care Unit with Sepsis. *Journal of Translational Medicine* 2009;7:1-9.

Klevens RM, Morrison MA, Nadle J, Petit S, Gershman K, Ray S, Harrison LH, Lynfield R, Dumyati G, Townes JM, Craig AS, Zell ER, Fosheim GE, McDougal LK, Carey RB, Fridkin SK. Invasive methicillin-resistant Staphylococcus aureus Infections in the United States. *Journal of the American Medical Association* 2007;298(15): 1763-1771.

Lampe F, Snyder S. Conversation with Michael Holick, PHD, MD: Vitamin D Pioneer. *Alternative Therapies* 2008;14(3):65-75.

Landrigan CP, Parry GJ, Bones CB, Hackbarth AD, Goldman DA, Sharek PJ. Temporal Trends in Rates of Patient Harm Resulting from Medical Care. *New England Journal of Medicine* 2010 Nov;363(22): 2124-2134.

Lee DM, Tajar A, Ulubaev A, Pendleton N. Association Between 25-hydroxyvitamin D levels, and cognitive Performance in Middle-aged and Older European Men. *Journal of Neurology, Neurosurgery, and Psychiatry* 2009;80:722-729.

Llewellyn DJ, Lang IA, Langa KM, Muniz-Terrera G, Phillips CL, Cherubini A, Ferruci L, Melzer D. Vitamin D and Risk of Cognitive Decline in

Elderly Persons. *The Archive of Internal Medicine* 2010 July 12;170 (13):1135-41.

Martineau AR, Wilkinson RJ, Wilkinson KA, Newton BK, Hall BM, Packe GE, Davidson RN, Eldridge SM, Maunsell ZJ, Rainbow SJ, Berry JL, Griffiths CJ. A Single Dose of Vitamin D Enhances Immunity to Mycobacteria. *American Journal of Respiratory and Critical Care Medicine* 2007;176:208-213.

Nishimura K, Shima M, Tsuqawa N, Matsumoto S, Harai h, santo Y, Nakajima S, Iwata M, Takaqi T, Kanda Y, Kanzaki T, Okano T, Ozono K. Long-term Hospitalization during Pregnancy is a Risk Factor for Vitamin D Deficiency in Neonates. *Journal of Bone Mineral Metabolism* 2003;21(2):103-8.

Nowson C. Nutritional Challenges for the Elderly. *Nutrition and Dietetics* 2007;64(4):S150-S155.

Sanders KM, Berk M, Pasco JA, Jacka FN. Association Between Depressive Symptoms and Vitamin D Deficiency in the Elderly. *Medical Hypothese* 2007;69(6):1316-1319.

Stokstad E. The Vitamin D Deficit. *Science* 2003;302(5652):6-10.

Sun X , Zemel MB. 1, 25-Dihydroxyvitamin D and Corticosteroid Regulate Adipocyte Nuclear Vitamin D Receptor. *International Journal of Obesity* 2008;32:1305-1311.

Sylvester B. Vitamin D Deficiency Impairs Daily Functioning in the Elderly. *Internal Medicine World Report* 2007;23.

Tiangga E, Gowda A, Dent JA. Vitamin D Deficiency in Psychiatric In-Patients and Treatment with Daily Supplements of Calcium and Ergocalciferol. *The Psychiatrist* 2008;32:390-393.

Valina-Toth AL B, Lai Z, Yoo W, Abou-Samra A, Gadegbeku CA, Flack JM. Relationship of Vitamin D and parathyroid Hormone with Obesity and Body Composition in African Americans. *Clinical Endocrinology* 2010;72(5):595-603.

Vanlint S, Nugent M, Durvasula S, Downs J, Leonard H. A Guide for the Assessment and Management of Vitamin D Status in People with Intellectual Disability. *Journal of Intellectual and Developmental Disability* 2008;33(2):184-188.

White JH. Vitamin D Signaling, Infectious Diseases, and Regulation of Innate Immunity. *Infection and Immunity* 2008;76(9):3837-3843.

Wilkins CH, Birge SJ, Sheline YI, Morris JC. Vitamin D Deficiency Affects Worse Cognitive Performance and Lower Bone Density in Older African Americans. *Journal of National Medical Association* 2009 April;101(4):349-54.

Yosipovitch G, Tang MBY. Practical Management of Psoriasis in the Elderly: The Use of Calcipotriol, a Vitamin D3 Analogue. *Drugs Aging* 2002;19(11):847-863.

Chapter Nine: Special Vitamin D Needs of Dark-Skinned Pregnant and Lactating Women and Dark-Skinned Children

Barnes MS, Robson PJ, Bonham MP, Strain JJ, Wallace JMW. Effect of Vitamin D Supplementation on Vitamin D Status and Bone Turnover Markers in Young Adults. *European Journal of Clinical Nutrition* 2006;60(6):727-733.

Barnevik–Olsson M, Gillberg C, Fernell E. Prevalence of Autism in Children born to Somali Parents Living in Sweden: A Brief Report. *Developmental Medicine and Child Neurology* 2010;50(8):598-601.

Beaver KM, Vaughn MG, Wright JP, DeLisi M, Howard MO. Three Dopaminergic Polymorphisms are Associated with Academic Achievement in Middle and High Schools. *Intelligence* 2010;38:596-604.

Bibuld D. Health Disparities and Vitamin D. *Clinical Reviews in Bone and Mineral Metabolism* 2009 April;7:63-76.

Bodnar LM, Simhan HN. Vitamin D may be a Link to Black-White Disparities in Adverse Birth Outcomes. *Obstetrics Gynecology Survey* 2010;65(4):273-284.

Bodnar LM, Krohn MA, Simhan HN. Racial and Seasonal Differences in 25-*Nutrition* Hydroxyvitamin D detected in Maternal Sera Frozen for over 40 years. *British Journal of Nutrition* 2009;1-1(2):278-84.

Bodnar LM, Simhan HN. Vitamin D may be a Link to Black-White Disparities in Adverse Birth Outcomes: Maternal Vitamin D deficiency Increases the Risk of Pre-eclampsia. *Journal ofClinical Endocrinology and Metabolism* 2007;92:3517-3522.

Bodnar LM, Wisner KL. Nutrition and Depression: Implications for Improving Mental Health among Childbearing-aged Women. *Biological Psychiatry* 2005;58(9):679-685.

Brehm JM, Celedón JC, Soto-Quiros ME, Avila L, Hunninghake GM, Forno E, Laskey D, Sylvia JS, Hollis BW, Weiss ST, Litonjua AA. Serum Vitamin D Levels and Markers of Severity of Childhood Asthma in Costa Rica. *American Journal of Respiratory and Critical Care Medicine* 2009;179:765-771.

Cui X, Pelekanos M, Burne TH, McGrath JJ, Eyles DW. Maternal Vitamin D Deficiency Alters the Expression of Genes involved in Dopamine Specification in the Developing Rat Mesencephalon. *Neuroscience Letter* 2010 Dec;486(3):220-223.

Dong Y, Stallmann-Jorgensen IS, Pollock NK, Harris RA, Keeton D, Huang Y, Li K, Bassali R, Guo D, Thomas J, Pierce GL, White J, Holick MF and Zhu H. A 16-Week Randomized Clinical Trial of of 2000 International Units Daily Vitamin D3 Supplementation in Black Youth:25-Hydroxyvitamin D, Adiposity, and Arterial Stiffness. *The Journal of Clinical Endocrinology and Metabolism* 2010;10:1210-1220.

Eyles D, Cui X, Pelekanos M, Kesby J, Burne T, Mcgrath J. S67-03 Developmental Vitamin D Deficiency (DVD) and Brain Dopamine Ontogeny. *European Psychiatry* 2009;24(1):S319-S330.

First BPA Detection in Infant Cord Blood: Study Found More than 200 Chemicals in Cord Blood of African American, Asian and Hispanic Newborns. *EWG Public Affairs* 2009;202:667-6982.

Freishtat RJ, Igbal SF, Pillai DK, Klein CJ, Ryan LM, Benton AS, Teach SJ. High Prevalence of Vitamin D Deficiency among Inner-City African American Youth with Asthma in Washington, DC. *The Journal of Pediatrics* 2010;156(6):948-952.

Gaggero M, Mariani L, Guarino R, Patrucco G, Ballardini G, Boscardini L, Barbaglia M, Bello L, Guala A. Vitamin D at Term of Pregnancy and During Lactation in White and Black Women Living in Northern Italy. *Minerva Ginecologica* 2010;62(2):91-96.

Grant WB. Official Recommended Intake for Vitamin D is Too Low: 2,000 IU/Day or More Needed for Optimal Health. *Orthomolecular Medicine News Service* 2010 February 19.

Hollis BW, Wagner CL. The Vitamin D Requirement During Human Lactation: The Facts and IOM's "Utter" Failure. *Public Health Nutrition* 2011 April;14(4):748-749.

Hypponen E, Hartikainen AL, Sovio U, Jarvelin MR, Pouta A. Does Vitamin D *Clinical* Supplementation in Infancy Reduce the Risk of Pre-eclampsia? *European Journal of Nutrition* 2007;61:1136-1139.

Kazemi A, Sharifi F, Jafari N, Mousavinasab N. High Prevalence of Vitamin D Deficiency Among Pregnant Women and their Newborns in an Iranian Population. *Journal of Women's Health* 2009;18(6):835-839.

Kesby JP, Cui X, Ko P, McGrath JJ, Burne THJ, Eyles DW. Developmental Vitamin D Deficiency Alters Dopamine Turnover in Neonatal Rat Forebrain. *Neuroscience Letters 2009;*461(2):155-158.

Lampe F, Snyder S. Conversation with Michael Holick, PHD. MD. Vitamin D Pioneer. Alternative *Therapies* 2008;14(3):65-75.

Linday LA, Umhua JC, Shindledecker RD, Dolitsky JN, Holick MF. Codliver Oil, the Ratio of Vitamin A and D, Frequent Respiratory Tract Infections, and Vitamin D Deficiency in Young Children in the United States. *Annals of Otology, Rhinology and Laryngology* 2010; 119(1):64-70.

Litonjua AA. Vitamin D and Asthma. *Respiratory Medicine* 2010;24(1):1-9.

McCacn JC, Bruce NA. Is there Convincing Biological or Behavioral Evidence Linking Vitamin D Deficiency to Brain Dysfunction? The FASEB Journal 2008;22:982-1001.

McGrath JJ, Eyles DW, Penderson CB. Neonatal Vitamin D Status and Risk of Schizophrenia. *Archive of General Psychiatry* 2010;67(9): 889-894.

McGrath JJ, Eyles DW, Mowry B, Yolken R, Buka S. Low Maternal Vitamin D as a Risk Factor for Schizophrenia: A Pilot Study Using Banked Sera. *Schizophrenia Research* 2003;63:73-78.

Mansbach JM, Ginde AA, Carmargo CA. Serum 25-hydroxyvitamin D Levels Among US Children Aged 1 to 11 Years: Do Children Need More Vitamin D? *Pediatrics* 2009 Nov;124:1404-10.

Merewood A, Mehta SD, Chen TC, Bauchner H, Holick MF. Association Between Vitamin D Deficiency and Primary Caesarean Section. *Journal of Clinical* Endocrinology and *Metabolism* 2008;94(3):940-945.

Parsons JP, Kaeding C, Phillips G, Jarjoura D, Wadley G, Mastronarde JG. Prevalence of Exercise-Induced Bronchospasm in a Cohort of Varsity College Athlete. *Medicine and Science in Sports and Exercise* 2007;39(9):1487-1492.

Rajakumar K, Fernstrom JD, Janosky JE, Greenspan SL. Vitamin D Insufficiency in Preadolescent African American Children. *Clinical Pediatrics* 2005;44:683-692.

Robinson CJ, Wagner CL, Hollis BW, Baatz JE, Johnson DD. Maternal Vitamin D and Fetal Growth In Early-onset Severe Preeclampsia. *American Journal of Obstetrics and Gynecology* 2011 March [Epub ahead of print].

Wagner CL, Taylor SN, Hollis BW. Does Vitamin D Make the World Go "Round"? *Breastfeeding Medicine* 2008 December;3(4):239-250.

Walker VP, Zhang X, Rastegar I, Liu PT, Hollis BW, Adams JS, Modlin RL. Cord Blood Vitamin D Status Impacts Innate Immune Responses. *Journal of Clinical Endocrinology Metabolism* 2011 April [Epub ahead of print].

Yu CKH, Sykes L, Sethi M, Teoh TG, Robinson S. Vitamin D Deficiency and Supplementation During Pregnancy. *Clinical Endocrinology* 2009; 70(5):685-690.

Chapter Ten: How Much Vitamin D Is Enough?

Boucher BJ. The 2010 Recommendations of the American Institute of Medicine for Daily Intakes of Vitamin. *Public Health Nutrition* 2011 April;14(4):740.

Brot C, Jorgensen NR, Sorensen OH. Smoking Reduces 25(OH)D Levels. *European Journal of Clinical Nutrition* 1999 December:53(12):920-926.

Cannell J, Era or Error? *Public Health Nutrition* 2011 April;14(4):743.

Fox J, Peters B, Prakash M, Arribas J, Hill A, Moecklinghoff C. Improvement in Vitamin D Deficiency Following Antiretroviral Regime Change: Results from the MONET Trial. *Aids Research Human Retroviruses* 2010;PMID:20854196.

Garland CF, French CB, Baggerly LL, Heaney RP. Vitamin D Supplement Doses and Serum 25- Hydroxyvitamin D in the Range Associated with Cancer Prevention. *Anticancer Research* 2011;31:607-612.

Grant WB. Is the Institute of Medicine Report on Calcium and Vitamin D good science? *Biological Research for Nurs*ing 2011 Apr;13(2):117-9.http://brn.sagepub.com/content/early/2011/01/10/1099800410 396947.long

Grant WB. The Institute of Medicine did not find the vitamin D-cancer link because it ignored Ultraviolet B Dose Studies. *Public Health Nutrition* 2011 April;14(4):745-746.

Grant WB, Holick MF. Benefits and Requirements of Vitamin D for Optimal Health: A Review. *Alternative Medicine Review* 2005; 10(2):94-105.

Grant WB. Official Recommended Intake for Vitamin D is Too Low: 2,000 IU/Day or More Needed for Optimal Health. *Orthomolecular Medicine News Service* 2010 February 19.

Heaney RP, Grant WB, Holick MF, Amling M. The IOM Report on Vitamin D Misleads. *Journal of Clininical Endocrinoly and Metabolism* eLetter; (4 March 2011) http://jcem.endojournals.org/cgi/eletters/ 96/1/53

Heaney RP, Holick MF. Why the IOM Recommendations for Ditamin D are Deficient. *Journal of Bone Mineral Research* 2011;26(3):455-457.

Heaney RP. Finding the Appropriate Referent for Vitamin D. Public Health Nutrition. 2011 April;14(4):749-750.

Holick MF. The D-batable Institute of Medicine Report: A D-lightful Perspective. Endocrine Practice 2011 Jan-Feb;17(1):143-149.

Holick MF. The IOM D-lemma. *Public Health Nutrition* 2011 May;14(5): 939-941

Lampe F, Snyder S. Conversation with Michael Holick, PHD, MD: Vitamin D Pioneer. Alternative *Therapies* 2008;14 (3): 65-75.

Mansbach JM, Ginde AA, Carmargo CA. Serum 25-hydroxyvitamin D Levels Among US Children Aged 1 to 11 Years: Do Children Need More Vitamin D? *Pediatrics* 2009 Nov; 124:1404-10.

Nurmi-Luthje I, Luthje P, Kaukonen J, Kataja M, Kuurne S, Naboulsi H, Karjalainen K. Post-Fracture Prescribed Calcium and Vitamin D Supplements Alone or, in Females With Concomitant Anti-Osteoporotic Drugs is Associated with Lower Mortality in Elderly Hip Fracture Patients: A Prospective Analysis. *Drugs and Aging* 2009;26(5):409-421.

Spreen A. Vitamin D conspiracy leads straight to Big Pharma. 02/19/2011   http://www.healthiertalk.com/vitamin-d-conspiracy-leads-straight-big-pharma-3396.

Stephenson DW, Peiris AN. The lack of vitamin D Toxicity with Megadoses of Daily Ergocalciferol (D2) Therapy: A Case Report and Literature Review. *Southern Medical Journal* 2009 July;102(7):765-768.

White JH. Vitamin D Signaling, Infectious Diseases, and Regulation of Innate Immunity. *Infection and Immunity* 2008;76(9):3837-3843.

Chapter Eleven: Exercise – An Essential Health Factor

Ardestani A, Parker B, Mathur S, Clarkson P, Pescatello LS, Hoffman HJ, Polk DM, Thompson PD. Relation of vitamin D level to maximum oxygen uptake in adults *American Journal of Cardiology* 2011 Feb; 107(8):1246-49.

Bartoszewska M, Kamboj M, Patel DR. Vitamin D, Muscle Function, and Exercise Performance. *Pediatric Clinics of North America* 2010 June;57(3):849-61.

Bell NH, Godsen RN, Henry DP, Shary J, Epstein S. The effects of Muscle-building Exercise on Vitamin D and Mineral Metabolism. *Journal of Bone Mineral Research* 2009 Aug;3(4):369-74.

Cannell JJ, Hollis BW, Sorenson MB, Taft TN, Anderson JJB. Athletic Performance and Vitamin D. *Medicine and Science in Sports and*

Exercise 2008 Oct; DOI:10.1249/MSS.0b01e3181930c2b:1102-1110.

Dowd J, Stafford, C. 2008. *The Vitamin D Cure.* New Jersey: John Wiley & Sons.

Gilsanz V, Kremer A, Mo AO, Wren T, Kremer R. Vitamin D Status and its relation to Muscle Mass and Muscle Fat in Young Women. *Journal of Clinical Endocrinology and Metabolism* 2010 Apr;95(4): 1595-1601.

Hamilton B. Vitamin D and Human Skeletal Muscle. *Scandinavian J of Medicine and Science in Sports* 2010 April;20(2):182-90.

Stewart JW, Alekel DL, Ritland LM, Van Loan M, Gertz E, Genschel U. Serum 25-hydroxyvitamin D is Related to Indicators of overall Physical Fitness in Healthy Postmenopausal Women. *Menopause* 2009 Nov-Dec;16(6):1093-101.

Chapters Twelve and Thirteen: Tips for Selecting and Preparing Foods and Fighting Inflammation with Anti-inflammatory Foods

Barker LA, Gout BS, Crowe TC. Hospital Malnutrition: Prevalence, Identification and Impact on Patients and the Healthcare System. *International Journal of Environmental Research and Public Health* 2011 Feb;8(2):514-527.

Chiuve SE, Korngold EC, Januzzi JL, Gantzer ML, Albert CM. Plasma and Dietary Magnesium And Risk of Sudden Cardiac Death in Women. *The American Journal of Clinical Nutrition* 2010 Nov;doi:10.3945.

Fallon S, Enig MG. 2001. *Nourishing Traditions: The Cookbook that Challenges Politically Correct Nutrition and the Diet Dictocrats.* Washington DC: New Trends Publishing.

Grant WB. Dietary Links to Alzheimer's Disease. *Alzheimer's Disease Review 2* 1997;42-55

Gardner EJ, Ruxton CHS, Leeds AR. Black Tea – Helpful or Harmful? A Review of the Evidence. *European Journal of clinical Nutrition* 2007 July;61(1)3-18.

Key TJ, Appleby PN, Spencer EA, Travis RC, Allen NE, Thorogood M, Mann JI. Cancer Incidence in British Vegetarians. *British Journal of Cancer* 2009;101:192-197.

Kita J. 9 Easy Ways to Clean Up Your Diet. *Prevention* 2010;62(3).

Li Y, Zang T, Korkaya H. et. Al. Sulforaphane, a Dietary Component of Broccoli/Broccoli Sprouts, Inhibits Breast Cancer Stem Cells. *Clinical Cancer Research* 2010;16(9):2580-90.

Paddock C. Organic Food Is More Nutritious Say EU Researchers. *Medical News Today* 2007 October.

Palmer S. Cultivate a Nutrient-Rich Approach to Eating for Life. *Environmental Nutrition* 2010.

Patel AV, Bernstein L, Deka A, Feigelson HS, Campbell PT, Gapstur SM, Colditz GA, Thun MJ. Leisure Time Spent Sitting in Relation to total Mortality in a Prospective Cohort of U.S. Adults. *American Journal of Epidemiology* 2010;172(4):419-429.

Rampersaud GC, Pereira MA, Girard BL, Adams J, Metzl JD. Breakfast habits, Nutritional Status, Body weight, and Academic Performance in Children and Adolescents. *Journal of American Dietetic Association* 2005 May;105(5):743-60.

Seyoum B, Seraj ES, Saenz C, Abdulkadir J. Hypomagnesemia in Ethiopians with Diabetes Mellitus. *Ethnicity and Disease* 2008 spring;18:147-151.

Yan J. Hyperactivity in Children Linked to Food Coloring. *Clinical and Research News* Nov 2007;42(19).

Zhang D, Al-Hendy M, Richard-Davis G, Montgomery-Rice V, Sharan C, Rajaratnam V, Khurana A, Al-Hendy A. Green Tea extract Inhibits Proliferation of Uterine Leiomyoma Cells in Vitro and in Nude Mice. *American Journal of Obstetrics and Gynecology* 2010 March;202(3):289.el-289.e9.

Index

About the Author

Emily Allison-Francis has an Associate Degree from the Jamaica School of Agriculture, a B.S. Degree in Nutrition from Tuskegee University in Alabama, an M.S. Degree in Nutrition from Hunter College of the City University of New York, an M.L.S. Degree in Library Science from Queens College of the City University of New York and a Post Graduate Diploma in Education from the University of the West Indies. Ms. Francis' many years of service in education, agriculture, nutrition and library science, include teaching high school agricultural science, chemistry and biology and working in a supervisory capacity with the Ministry of Education in Jamaica, Caribbean. Prior to serving at the Ministry of Education, she worked at the Ministry of Agriculture in Jamaica, guiding rural farm families in matters related to food production and nutrition. Ms. Francis has taught biology, earth science, food and nutrition, food preparation skills, and library research skills to high school students during her years of teaching with the New York City Department of Education. She writes articles for newspapers in the New York City area and worked as an adjunct professor and reference librarian at Medgar Evers College of the City University of New York. She provides nutrition workshops for community organizations and is an ardent advocate for holistic health education and preventive health care.

Visit her website at www.healthieryounutrition.com